MW01143410

COLLINS GEM
CRICKET

a mine of information

COLLINS GEM
DIETING

a mine of information

COLLINS GEM
DOGS

a mine of information

COLLINS GEM
FIRST AID

a mine of information

COLLINS GEM
INTERNET
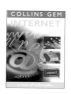
a mine of information

COLLINS GEM
PREDICTING

a mine of information

COLLINS GEM
Ready
REFERENCE

a mine of information

COLLINS GEM
SHARKS

a mine of information

COLLINS GEM
WHALES
& DOLPHINS
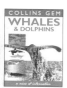
a mine of information

COLLINS GEM
WHISKY

a mine of information

COLLINS GEM
WORD
PROCESSING
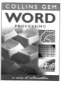
a mine of information

COLLINS GEM
Your PC

a mine of information

COLLINS GEM

CHILDCARE

Belinda Grant Viagas

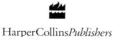

HarperCollins*Publishers*

Belinda Grant Viagas (ND, DO DipC) is the author of Natural Healthcare for Women, Pocket A–Z of Natural Healthcare, Detox Diet Book **and** Natural Remedies for Common Ailments. **She also writes for various health magazines.**

NOTE: *All information in this book has been fully checked and approved by experienced medical and paramedical staff. However, this book is not intended to be a substitute for professional medical care. It should only be used as a guide to actions that may be needed prior to obtaining professional help.*

HarperCollins Publishers
Westerhill Rd, Bishopbriggs, Glasgow G64 2QT

Created and produced by
Grapevine Publishing Services, London

First published 2000
Reprint 10 9 8 7 6 5 4 3 2 1 0

© Grapevine Publishing Services Ltd, 2000

Photography by Christina Jansen
Illustrations by David Mostyn

ISBN 0 00 472468 2

Printed in Italy by Amadeux S.p.A.

Contents

Introduction 6

Preparing for your baby 7
Joining the family 10
Your baby's development 11
New babies 12
Premature babies 13
The first six months 14
Six months to one year 15
One year to 18 months 17
Eighteen months to three years 18
Toddler to pre-school 20

A–Z of Childcare 21

Adoption and fostering 22
Allergies 23
Artificial respiration 24
Asthma 25
Bathing babies and
  children 26
Bedwetting 28
Bonding 30
Bottle-feeding 31
Breast-feeding 33
Bronchitis 36
Bruises 37
Bullying 37
Burns 39
Car journeys 40
Car safety 41
Cardiac massage 42
Catarrh 43
Check-ups 44
Chickenpox 47
Childminders 48
Choking 49
Circumcision 50
Colds 51
Colic 52
Comfort behaviours 53
Concussion 54
Constipation 54

Conversation	55	Friendships	95
Cot death	55	Genitals	97
Coughs	57	Gifted children	98
Cradle cap	58	Glandular fever	99
Crawling	59	Glue ear	100
Croup	60	Growth	100
Crying	61	Hand-eye	
Cuts	62	co-ordination	102
Diarrhoea	63	Handicaps	103
Disability	64	Hay fever	104
Discipline	65	Head injuries	105
Dressing babies and		Hearing	106
children	67	Hiccups	108
Drinking liquids	69	Holidays	109
Drowning	70	Hospital stays	111
Dummies	71	Hygiene	113
Earache	73	Hyperactivity	114
Eating problems	74	Immunization	115
Eczema	76	Independence	116
E numbers	77	Insomnia	117
Eyesight	77	Left- or	
Falls	79	right-handedness	118
Fears	80	Lying	119
Fever	81	Manual skills	120
Fever fits	82	Manners	121
Fighting	83	Massage	122
First aid	85	Mealtimes	124
First foods	90	Measles	126
Fontanelles	93	Meningitis	127
Fractures	94	Moodiness	128

Mouth-to-mouth resuscitation	129	Sore throat	159
Mumps	129	Speech	160
Nappies	130	Stammering	162
Nappy rash	133	Sticky eye	163
Nosebleeds	133	Stings	163
Nutrition	134	Stomach ache	164
Only children	135	Suffocation	165
Pets	136	Sunburn	165
Playing	138	Swallowed objects	167
Post-natal depression	139	Swimming	169
Potty training	139	Teething and caring for teeth	170
Rashes	141	Temper tantrums	172
Reading and writing	142	Temperature	174
Routine	143	Thumb-sucking	175
Rubella	144	Toys	176
Safety	145	Travel sickness	178
Separation anxiety	147	Twins	180
Sex differences	148	Urinary tract infections	182
Shoes	149	Vaccinations	183
Shyness	150	Vomiting	186
Sibling rivalry	151	Walking	187
Sleep patterns	153	Weaning	188
Sleeping problems	154	Whooping cough	189
Slow learners	157	Worms	191
Smacking	158		

Useful addresses   **192**

Introduction

Congratulations. Now that you have just had a baby, or brought a child into your home, your life will never be the same again. All sorts of practical changes will take place and existing relationships will alter dramatically. Caring for babies and children is a great responsibility, yet it is also one that is incredibly fulfilling.

All children have their own personality and humour, with differing needs, wants and responses. Even identical twins will have different character traits. Your child is and will be unique, and your own responses will depend on his or her personality regardless of changing fashions in the more practical aspects of childcare, such as whether or not to use a

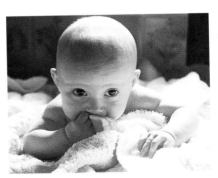

playpen or dummies, and whether to choose breast- or bottle-feeding. Learning to trust your own love and instincts is all-important in caring for your children. Alongside this, practical parenting classes offer a wealth of information to guide new parents, and there is also much to be gained from sifting through the wisdom and experience of older family members and friends with children.

Motherhood brings its own challenges, and it is important that you care for your own health as well as that of your baby. The relationship with your partner, and their relationship with the baby will all come under the spotlight, as will issues surrounding routine and the division of chores in the home. Previously simple things like shopping and cooking will suddenly cease to be quite so simple and may have to be reorganized or rethought.

PREPARING FOR YOUR BABY

Before your baby arrives you should try to discuss and make decisions about some fundamental issues:

- Do you want your baby to sleep in the bed with you? Advice varies considerably. However, it is recommended that your baby sleeps in the same room as you. There are special cots that can be adapted to fit next to your bed, so that the baby is close to you. Try to change rooms and furniture around well before the baby arrives, because this is when you will have the time and energy. It is also especially important if there are other children in the home, as it gives them time to adjust to the new arrangements before the baby's arrival.

- Who will be responsible for your baby's primary care? Agree now as far as possible on who will be expected to take time off work if your child is ill, for example. What sort of support will you get from friends and family members? It is never too early to enlist baby-sitters.

- What will be your position on discipline?

Before long you will also need to take practical measures to baby-proof your home (*see also* **Safety**). It may seem a bit early to undertake this sort of work, but your baby will be crawling before very long, and will have an amazing curiosity about his world. Try getting down to floor level yourself to see what is accessible from there – what can be reached, pulled on, climbed up, whether there are any sharp edges there, or things that look especially interesting from that angle.

Go through every room in turn, making sure that you address as many safety features as you possibly can. Get into the habit of turning pan handles inwards when you are cooking, not using tablecloths (these can be pulled on, bringing all the table's contents down with them), clearing sharp tools and utensils away immediately after use, keeping medicines and cleaning products well out of reach. If you have a garden, you will need to do a safety check there too. Among the first words to teach your child will be strong commands such as 'no' or 'hot'. This should be sharp enough to stop him in his tracks.

Essentials for your newborn

- six all in one stretchsuits
- six vests or bodysuits
- two cardigans or jackets
- a shawl
- a sun hat or warm hat depending on time of year
- a snowsuit for the winter
- scratch mittens
- socks and booties
- more nappies than you think you will need
- baby wipes/cotton wool
- a crib or cot with waterproof sheets, fitted sheets and blankets
- an appropriate car seat, properly installed (preferably by an experienced fitter)
- pram/pushchair
- changing mat and bag
- towels and face flannels
- baby comb, hairbrush and nail scissors or clippers

If you are bottle-feeding, you will also need sterilizing equipment, a bottle brush and at least six bottles with teats.

Taking a first aid course may also be a good idea, and it is important to keep yourself feeling fit, possibly adopting a new fitness or exercise regime.

JOINING THE FAMILY

If you have other children in the home, the arrival of a new baby may require even more careful preparation:

- Involve older children as much as possible – give them some responsibility for showing off the baby to visitors, for example.

- Consider whether they should continue with their usual routine, or perhaps take some time off from nursery to be around you and at home.

- Encourage everyone, including visitors, to make a fuss of your existing child or children as well as admiring the new baby.

- Show your children how to handle the baby, taking care when lifting him, and supporting his head, and let them know when they will be able to do that – i.e. make rules about handling and playing with the new baby, perhaps

TRAINING YOUR PETS

If you have pets, teach them before the birth to stay out of the bedrooms, and preferably out of the kitchen too. Make sure they will respond to a strong command of 'no', 'leave', or 'down'. Have your animal checked for fleas, worms and infections, and spend some time introducing it to other children. Never leave your baby or infant alone with your pet. (*See also* **Pets**)

limiting it to when a parent is around for younger children. Try to awaken your child's protective instincts by explaining just how fragile and vulnerable the new baby is.

YOUR BABY'S DEVELOPMENT

When your baby is born, he will be given a medical assessment to ensure that all is well. After that, it is important to keep a check on his development, and his size and weight, through regular clinic check-ups and home visits which will also give you an opportunity to raise any concerns you may have. All parents are anxious about their baby's wellbeing, particularly if it's their first, but routine tests and measurements will reassure you that all is going well.

NEW BABIES

Within five minutes of being born, your baby will be medically checked and assessed. Observations will be made on the following:

• *Appearance* – to check for birthmarks, condition of the skin, and that everything is in place. The baby's head will often look out of shape or somewhat out of proportion. This is a normal response to its journey through the birth canal, and you may notice specific indentations or marks if forceps or suction were used. These will disappear and should cause no concern.

• *Pulse* – to ensure that there is a steady heartbeat, and that the process of being born has not been overtaxing.

• *Cry* – to clear the lungs, or demonstrate a response to stimulation. This is an initial check on the integrity of the nervous system.

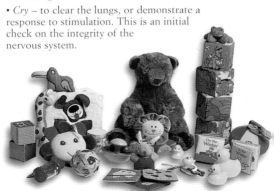

• *Muscle tone* – to check for physical integrity and that the limbs are free and flexible.

• *Respiration* – to check that the baby's respiratory system is working effectively.

Your baby will also have certain characteristic responses:

• *his grasp* – newborn babies curl their fingers around whatever is placed in their hands;

• *stepping* – if a newborn baby is held up, supported under the arms, and 'stood' on a firm surface, he will appear to be taking steps;

• *response to sudden noise or other frights* – new babies tend to arch their backs and reach out with their arms as if looking for someone to cling to for protection.

PREMATURE BABIES

Premature babies (i.e. those born before 37 weeks of gestation) need extra care, possibly involving medical intervention. They may not be brought home to the family until they are older and stronger but most hospitals allow mothers to stay in with the baby for as long as they are able, or to visit as often as they wish.

The earlier a baby is born, the less time he will have had to develop. Some of the more common problems in premature babies include the need for extra help with breathing because the lungs are not fully functional, and an absent or poorly developed sucking reflex which can cause feeding problems. Premature babies also find it even harder than other babies to regulate their temperature, and can become cold extremely quickly. Their immature immune system makes them more prone to infections. Your midwife and hospital will advise on any special care required.

THE FIRST SIX MONTHS

Newborns have no real control over their movements, and their neck muscles are not developed enough to hold the head up. Vision is mainly blurred; they can see best if the object is not more that 25 cm away and objects with starkly contrasting colours, like black and white, will catch their attention.

Early smiles are likely to be an indication of wind, because control of the facial muscles develops quite slowly. Crying is the main means of a new baby's communication, and it will take a while for this to differentiate into cries that indicate hunger, discomfort, etc. As the months progress, he will be more easily distracted, and will often turn towards a familiar voice, and stop crying in order to listen to it. By about four months, your baby will hold his head up and turn it. He will be able to sit up with support for up to half an hour at a time, and will also begin to make cooing and other sounds in his throat. He will start to spend more time awake between feeds.

Your baby's second check-up with a doctor should be at around eight weeks. He will be physically examined, and you will be able to discuss any questions you may have. You will also be invited to the surgery to have your baby immunized: at two, three and four months you will be offered the first course of combined vaccines against diphtheria, tetanus, pertussis (whooping cough), HiB (a cause of meningitis and pneumonia) and poliomyelitis (*see also* **Vaccinations**).

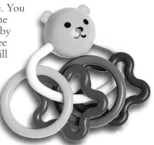

SIX MONTHS TO ONE YEAR

Between six and eight months your baby should be sitting up with a straight back, and may be able to sit on his own. He will take some of his own weight when standing, and will respond to you physically in a host of ways like raising his arms up towards you in order for you to lift him. He may also be using his arms to pull himself up, or to reach for things. He will be learning to crawl – forwards or backwards!

Objects and people will tend to be of equal interest in your baby's short attention span, although he will respond quickly to familiar people and voices. He will be exploring using different grips, and putting everything into his mouth, including his feet. He will begin to imitate sounds and to laugh, and will respond to different tones of voice. By about six months your baby will respond to his name.

Hand clapping and games like peek-a-boo will interest your baby. Repetition is a source of great pleasure; and babies find definite ways to let you know if they are cross. This is why, for instance, your baby might become rigid and scream or throw his head back when you want to feed or change him when he would rather be exploring or playing at something else. He will also begin to discriminate, around now, between his primary care giver and other people. This can be a trying time, particularly to those 'out of favour', but it is important to your baby's development.

At around six months, your baby will have a simple hearing test called a distraction test, at the clinic or at your doctor's surgery. This is a rudimentary procedure, but can pick up potential problems and alert the medical staff to provide early help before the baby's development is affected. This is also an opportunity for you to discuss your baby's general development, and any concerns you may have.

BABY CLOTHES

Babies grow very quickly and soon outgrow their first clothes. They also tend to leak from both ends, however, and need frequent changes of clothing. Hand-me-down clothes from friends or family are therefore very useful in the early days, and will save you lots of money.

The measles, mumps and rubella (German measles) combined vaccine is offered when your baby is over a year old (*see also* **Vaccinations**).

ONE YEAR TO 18 MONTHS

By around 15 months your baby may well be walking and will be confident standing alone. He will creep up stairs on his hands and knees and creep back down again very slowly, backwards. His manual skills will have improved too and he may be able to place one brick on top of another.

By the time your baby is 18 months old, he will have learned an amazing amount, and will have perfected an enormous number of skills and types of movement. He will be moving around on his own, often quite safely (without bumping into things), and will be able to carry something like a favourite toy with him. He will be good at climbing, and will have attained a sense of balance, enabling him to bend over to pick things up without toppling. He will be able to pick up small objects, and will make round scribbles with a pen or colouring pencil (*see also* **Hand–eye co-ordination**). He will be noticing moving objects in the middle distance.

His speech may be almost recognizable, in that he may string together groups of familiar sounds, but he may not use more than a dozen true words. Understanding is good, and he will follow simple conversations and instructions. His attention span is still short, but he will be pointing at things and

vocalizing his desire for them. He will enjoy 'singing'
and music.

He will probably want to feed himself, enjoying the
mess this will make, and he will begin to copy and
learn from your actions – whether it's hoovering or
sitting back with a sigh. He will probably want to be in
your company, but should be happy to play on his own
so long as you remain in view.

18 MONTHS TO THREE YEARS

Muscle control is developing and your baby will know
when he has filled a nappy, and may even know
beforehand that he wants to. If so, this is a potty-
training cue for you, although 18 months is about the
earliest you would want to begin this.

At around 18 months
your child will have a
further develop-
ment assessment
with your doctor
or health visitor.
This will
often

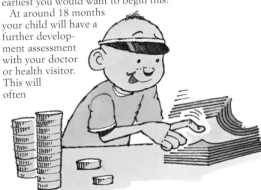

be as simple as watching your child at play, and confirming that basic skills are being attained. Again, there will be an opportunity for you to discuss any concerns or questions you may have regarding your child's development.

By the age of three your child will be walking up and down stairs quite safely on his own, and will be able to achieve feats of balance and co-ordination like walking on tiptoe, standing on one foot and possibly hopping. Drawing skills will have developed to reproducing recognizable objects, even faces, and your child will enjoy naming and matching colours to use. He will be using paintbrushes, and may even be able to cut things with children's scissors. His creativity will be developing at a dashing pace.

He should be familiar with the concept of numbers, although not necessarily very accurate in his counting. He will have his own favourite stories, nursery rhymes and songs or prayers, and may be able to repeat them on his own. He will be making himself understood verbally, most of the time at least, and will be asking questions about everything, regardless of whether he understands the answers. He will enjoy 'helping' you, and will be able to play using make-believe.

Toilet control should be good by three years, but he might not make it through the night without accidents and may need to be reminded to go, especially when other exciting things are happening.

At this stage your child will remember everything he sees and hears, and will be liable to repeat it. He may be losing any wariness of strangers, so this is a time to teach good safety techniques (*see also* **Safety**), and make these part of his social understanding.

You will be offered the booster diphtheria and tetanus combined vaccine, and polio; and the second dose of the MMR immunization three years after the first course was completed (*see also* **Vaccinations**).

TODDLER TO PRE-SCHOOL

Social skills become the focus of your child's learning, and making friends and being with other children will enable him to learn a lot about early negotiation skills and the art of compromise, as well as practical sharing and improved co-ordination.

Conversation skills will now be quite advanced, and will include the ability to listen and respond. Curiosity about others needs to be developed, and children who have been at home with their parents until now should be prepared for school by introducing them to other adults and children, and letting them feel part of a larger group.

AN A–Z OF CHILDCARE

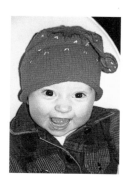

Adoption and fostering

Many people nowadays choose to adopt or foster children. While adopting a child means taking on the full mantle of parent, the role of foster parent or 'carer' varies according to the age of the child and the length of time he stays with the family. A stay may be as short as just a few weeks or may last for years with varying degrees of emotional involvement.

Adopted children often feel an extra need for reassurance, particularly where other siblings are involved. There are arguments for not telling a child that he is adopted until he is much older, although current thinking is in favour of telling the child just as soon as he is able to understand.

Great care is taken when choosing parents for adoption and fostering. Factors such as age (there is often an age limit of 35 for a woman and 40 for a man) are amongst those considered in a full screening and assessment process. Some local authority organizations only consider applications from people living locally, while other agencies may specialize in finding families of a particular race or religious faith. People choosing overseas adoption are subject to the same rigorous assessment guidelines, and there are inevitably additional paperwork and complications involved.

Advice on fostering and adoption is available through your healthcare advisor, and through the local social services department. Private services are also available.

Allergies

Allergies can be caused by anything from cows' milk to animal fur, peanuts, insect stings, pollen, chemicals (in soap powders, for example), or house dust mites' droppings found in bedding and soft furnishings. Reactions vary from child to child, and will depend on the substance they are reacting to, and the state of their immune system. Allergies often run in families. Typical symptoms can include asthma, eczema, diarrhoea, cold-type symptoms, constant mucus congestion and skin rashes and irritation.

Sometimes the trigger is obvious, if the rash appears immediately after your child has stroked the cat, for example. Other causes may require a bit of investigative work. If you think your child may be allergic but you're not sure of the allergen, it would be a good start to keep a food diary, in which you note down everything your child eats and when symptoms appear. This should enable you to spot any connections between certain foods and your child's reactions. If you suspect a food or food group, remove it from your child's diet for one week, and see if his symptoms improve. Never remove more than one food at a time, and seek specialist advice if you uncover an allergy to a major food group such as wheat or dairy produce as you will need to compensate nutritionally for foods being removed long term.

Vacuum regularly to keep your home as free as possible of airborne irritants and dust mites, particularly if the source of your child's allergy is as yet unknown; and choose synthetic soft furnishings, pillows and bedding. Place soft toys in a plastic bag and put in the freezer overnight once a month to kill off any dust mites.

> Peanuts can cause a life-threatening allergic reaction in some children. The most common symptoms are:
>
> - sudden, sharp stomach pain
> - swelling of the face, lips and tongue
> - difficulty in breathing
> - shock
>
> Parents of children with a peanut allergy must be extra vigilant when checking food labels. They may be given pre-loaded syringes so that they can give immediate treatment in case of a reaction.

See also **Asthma, Hay fever, Stings**

Artificial respiration
See **First aid**

Asthma

More than one child in ten develops asthma at some stage, and correct diagnosis and treatment are essential. Symptoms include wheezing and shortness of breath, and a dry cough. Asthma may be caused by a number of factors from pollution to allergies or even emotional upsets. There is a strong genetic link. Symptoms also worsen during coughs and colds, or in areas of damp, and of high atmospheric pollution (e.g. most cities, and on main traffic routes).

In the event of an asthma attack, stay calm and seek medical attention as quickly as possible. If your child is already taking medication, be sure to show it to the medical staff. Treatment may include taking medicine and using a ventilator or inhaler to relieve attacks.

Some asthma sufferers find that their physical activities are restricted. Sudden exertion and prolonged strenuous exercise may need to be avoided but regular gentle exercise will strengthen your child's health and improve his fitness. It is important to let carers and teachers know of your child's condition, and about any medication he may need to take. The good news is that more than half of asthmatic children grow out of it completely by the age of 21.

Measures that will help asthma sufferers include:
- keeping pets outdoors as much as possible to mini-mize shedding of animal hair around the house

- dusting all surfaces regularly and boiling bedding at least once a week
- buying mattresses, duvets and pillows with special hypo-allergenic covers and fillings
- never exposing your child to cigarette smoke
- hoovering regularly with an airtight system
- enclosing soft toys in a plastic bag in the freezer overnight once a month to kill off any house dust mites.

See also **Allergies**

Bathing babies and children

Babies do not need to be bathed every day; two or three times a week will suffice if you 'top and tail' in between. You will need the following equipment to bath your baby:

- a baby bath, or a towel to wrap around the taps in the sink

- a big soft towel

- a small bowl of boiled, cooled water

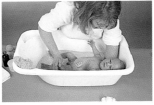

- cotton wool and a flannel
- shampoo and/or soap (though not for babies under six weeks)
- clean clothes and a nappy

Make sure the room you will be bathing the baby in is warm, and that the water in the bath is blood heat (29.4° C or 85° F). Test that it is not too hot, using your elbow or the inside of your wrist. Before undressing the baby, dip some cotton wool into the bowl of water, and use it to clean his eyes, ears and nose. Never use cotton buds to push inside – soft moistened cotton wool will work just as well and be safer. You will also need to wash around the umbilical area in new babies.

Once he is undressed, place one arm around your baby's shoulders, supporting the head, and your other arm under one leg to support his bottom, and lower him slowly into the warm water. Still holding the baby's head and shoulders securely with one hand, use your other hand to wash him all over. Babies of under six weeks old should not be washed with soap at all, and even after that, an oatmeal bag is an equally good cleanser, and can be especially useful if there are any skin complaints. Wash the hair last, using the flannel to rinse with, and make sure that no shampoo runs forward into the baby's eyes. Lift the baby out carefully by slipping one hand underneath his bottom, placing him directly on to a soft towel.

You might prefer to take your baby into the bath

> **Caution:** Never leave your baby unattended in the water for even a few seconds. Babies can drown in only a small amount of water. Even toddlers should not be left alone in a bath.

with you as long as the water is not too hot or deep, although it is probably best to make sure that someone else is around to hold him while you are getting in and out of the bath to avoid the danger of slipping.

As your child gets older he will enjoy playing with floating toys and containers in the bath – empty shampoo bottles are fine. Bath time will become a fun time and it is also a good way of establishing an evening routine.

See also **Routine**

Bedwetting

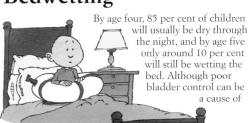

By age four, 85 per cent of children will usually be dry through the night, and by age five only around 10 per cent will still be wetting the bed. Although poor bladder control can be a cause of bedwetting, more often it is a sign of some form of upset or stress. Relapses often occur when a new baby is brought into the home, or when starting school, or in response to some other major event.

Patience and understanding are important when dealing with this problem. Do not make a fuss when changing sheets (older children may prefer to do this themselves), and make a point of finding time to discuss the situation and listen to your child's views.

If bedwetting is a recurrent problem, a waterproof undersheet is a good idea. There are also alarms on the market that sound a gentle buzzer when the child begins to wet, and this should be enough to wake them. Other tips include:

- encouraging older children not to drink for two hours before bed (with toddlers this may not be worth the aggravation it would cause)
- making sure your child goes to the toilet before bed
- ensuring windows are tightly closed on rainy nights
- checking internal plumbing – the sound of running water can encourage urinating
- keeping the child warm (but don't use an electric blanket – choose hot water bottles instead).

Check with your GP if bedwetting persists as there may be an underlying physical cause.

Bonding

'Bonding' usually arises naturally out of a parent's desire to care for a new baby, but it is not necessarily an instantaneous reaction as soon as they set eyes on their baby. For many parents bonding is a process that grows over time.

The chemical and hormonal changes that occur around birth predispose many mothers to bond with their baby, and the baby's response is automatic, although it may yet be some time before they can recognize their mother by sight. Early recognition is often through smell and occurs at a chemical level.

Some women experience difficulty in bonding with their baby. This may be because of unforeseen delivery problems, a premature or handicapped baby that is taken into a special care unit, feeding problems or even sheer exhaustion. However, it is important to raise feelings of detachment with your doctor as soon as possible as they can be a sign of **post-natal depression** (*see* page 139).

Fathers, too, need time to bond, and the more contact they have with their baby early on, the better. For their part, babies and children will also bond with other prime carers and significant people in their lives, such as grandparents or members of their extended family who spend a lot of time with them.

Feeding times provide a good opportunity to establish and then deepen the bond between parents and baby. This is a time when you can establish eye-contact, and be exclusively available to them. Other activities that will enable you to reinforce the bond include bathing, nappy changing, play, massage or simply falling off to sleep together. As your child grows, the things you do together will change, but even time spent learning the alphabet or singing songs will continue to draw you closer together.

Once established, the bond can be very strong, and partings become painful for both parents and child. It is important that you allow your child to become independent from you as soon as he is ready. Ultimately, this will strengthen the bond between you.

See also **Massage, Separation anxiety**

Bottle-feeding

If you are planning to bottle-feed your baby you will need:

- at least six bottles and teats
- a supply of formula milk
- sterilizing equipment (*see page 33*)
- a bottle brush.

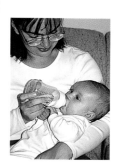

There are a number of different formula milks on the market. You will need to choose the one best suited to your requirements – whether you are exclusively bottle-feeding or switching to a bottle after weeks or months of breast-feeding. Your midwife or health visitor should be able to help you with your choice, taking into account age and any allergies that run in the family.

Always follow the instructions for making up feeds closely, making sure that the proportions are correct. Formula is harder for your baby to digest than breast-milk, so be patient and be prepared for a change in routines, as well as some minor digestive upsets.

Sit in a comfortable position with your baby held close to you; there is no reason why bottle-feeding should be any less of a 'bonding' experience than breast-feeding. Tilt the bottle so that the teat fills with milk, and then slip this into your baby's mouth. Keep the bottle tilted while you are feeding to prevent air from entering the teat. Allow for a few breaks in a feed when you can 'wind' the baby. This is most easily done by lifting him on to your shoulder, and gently rubbing or patting him on the back. Resume feeding, but never force your baby to empty the bottle.

Your baby may become thirsty between feeds, and you can give him some cooled, boiled water in a sterilized bottle. As you learn to distinguish his cries, it will be easier to tell when he is thirsty. Following a schedule will introduce routine that your baby will gain security from, but you may feel that feeding on demand is more appropriate. Choose a system that's convenient for you as well and adapt it as he grows older and his needs change.

STERILIZING

Bottles and all other equipment used for feeding your baby will need to be regularly sterilized. This can be done using any of the following:

- sterilizing tablets or liquid, which can be bought from the chemist
- an electric steamer
- the hot cycle in a dishwasher (at least 80° C/ 175° F); but not all teats are dishwasher safe so always check first
- a microwave bottle sterilizer.

Breast-feeding

Although not everybody can or wants to breast-feed, it is generally recognized as being best for both mother and child. It conveys your natural immunity to your child, and is an excellent way to 'bond' with your baby. Make sure, however, that it is your decision, and that

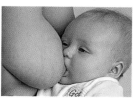

you are happy with it. If you are embarrassed about breast-feeding in public places, you may find it helpful to wear loose, baggy clothing that allows you to feed discreetly. Meeting with other breast-feeding mothers can also help to make you feel more relaxed and many shops and public places now provide 'mothers' rooms' for women who prefer privacy when feeding.

Advantages of breast-feeding:

- breast milk is naturally designed for your baby
- breast milk contains antibodies which help him to fight infections
- breast milk is easily digested and absorbed
- it is easy and practical – always available and at the right temperature
- breast-fed babies are less likely to develop allergies
- very tiny, premature babies are more likely to thrive on breast milk

---

Be patient with yourself and with your baby when you start breast-feeding. It will take you both a little while to get used to it. Start each feed on alternate breasts so that both are equally stimulated, which should help to prevent engorgement. In the early weeks try to follow cues from your baby. Feed when he 'asks' to be fed and for as long as he wants. He will show that he has finished by either letting go of the breast, or falling asleep. As he gets older, try to feed only when he is hungry, not just for comfort.

Bear in mind that what you eat will influence your milk so try to avoid very heavily spiced foods as well as a large intake of caffeine or alcohol. Avoid drugs as far as possible (although you may need to take painkillers for some breast-feeding problems), and make sure your doctor or pharmacist knows you are breast-feeding before they prescribe any medication.

The maternity hospital and/or your health centre may run breast-feeding support groups where you can share your experiences or any problems with other mothers. Your midwife/health visitor should also be able to offer help and advice.

Once you have breast-feeding well under way (usually around six weeks) you may want to start expressing milk to give the baby later by bottle. The most efficient way to do this is using a breast pump. Advantages of this include:

- giving your partner an opportunity to feed the baby
- allowing you some freedom
- getting your baby used to taking a bottle.

Twins can be breast-fed successfully and both can be fed at the same time (although you may choose to feed them separately at first until feeding is well established). Your milk supply will increase to meet the extra demand, but you may need help with the logistics to begin with.

Some women choose to breast-feed exclusively for six months, but this is a very individual choice, and other foods may be introduced before this.

See also **Bottle-feeding, First foods, Weaning**

Bronchitis

This is an inflammation of the airways which is often caused by a bacterial or viral infection. Symptoms include rapid and wheezy breathing, and a dry cough that worsens as the chest becomes more congested. There may be yellow or greenish phlegm, and symptoms are often worse at night when there may also be vomiting. Encourage your child to cough up and spit out any phlegm rather than swallowing it, and keep an eye on his temperature. Give him lots to drink to ensure he does not become dehydrated, and keep him still as far as possible to conserve his energy.

During coughing attacks place young children across your knee and pat their back to help expel mucus. If breathing becomes difficult, use steam inhalations to help clear the chest, and place a bowl of boiled water next to the bed, to which you have added one drop of eucalyptus essential oil. Keep your child warm, but if he develops a mild fever wash him down with tepid water to cool him. If symptoms worsen or do not improve, consult your doctor; if the infection is bacterial in origin a course of antibiotics may be needed.

> **Caution:** Always consult your doctor if you suspect bronchitis. If you notice a blue tinge around the lips or mouth, or if breathing becomes laboured, take your child to your GP or to hospital straight away as he may be in need of oxygen.

Bruises

Bruising is a discoloration of the skin caused by broken blood vessels. Sometimes there will also be a small bump. Most bruises do not need any treatment, but a cold compress held in place for about ten minutes may limit any swelling. This can be a clean tea-towel held under the cold tap, then wrung out and applied like a bandage, or a bag of frozen peas or some ice wrapped in a towel.

Ensure there is plenty of vitamin C in your child's diet as this may help to reduce bruising.

> **Caution:** If the pain caused by the bruise worsens after 24 hours, or if it has not begun to fade after a few days, consult your doctor. Also watch out for bruising for no apparent reason. Both may be signs of more serious conditions.

Bullying

If you notice a general change in your child's demeanour and learning ability, or a reluctance to go to school or nursery, it may be that he is being bullied. It is important to take action straight away, because in severe cases, bullying can permanently damage a child's self-esteem and even affect his immune system and his future health and wellbeing.

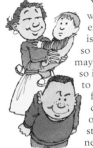

You should always comfort a child who is suffering from bullies, and encourage him to tell you about what is happening. A bullied child can feel so undermined by these attacks that he may not have the confidence to complain, so it is important to make it easy for him to talk to you and explain how he is feeling about it. Often, informing the child's teacher, minder, or the parent of the bullying child will be enough to stop these attacks, but you may also need to discuss with them what action is to be taken, or even to separate your child from the bullies in some more definite way. Always support your child, and reinforce his self-esteem and security.

With older children, discuss strategies for coping with incidents should they happen again. For example, self-defence classes run specifically for children can provide the necessary confidence and assertiveness to deal with difficult situations. In every case, remind your child that he must ask for help from the nearest authority as soon as he feels he is being bullied and encourage him to fight back only as a last resort.

If bullying persists, contact an advice line such as Childline (tel: 0800 1111) or ask your GP to refer you for specialized help.

See also **Discipline, Fighting**

Burns

Take immediate action in the event of any burn.

If your child has a heat burn from touching a flame or hot substance, try to cool the affected area. Run it under the cold tap, or apply an ice pack. Do this for at least ten minutes to reduce the heat thoroughly. Then take the child to hospital.

If your child's clothing is on fire, place him on the floor and either douse the flames with water or smother them with a heavy blanket. Remove smouldering clothing but do not attempt to peel away material that is sticking to the skin.

For an electrical burn, turn off the power. If this is not possible push your child away from the power source using a broom handle, cushion, newspaper or any other non-metallic object. Cool the area of any localized burn, and take the child to hospital.

Chemical burns need to be treated differently. Remove any soaked clothing if you can, run plenty of cold water over the affected area, and then cover the burn with a clean cloth. Take a sample of the offending chemical with you to the hospital.

Scalds (burns caused by steam or boiling liquid) should be treated in the same way as ordinary burns, by cooling the affected area under the cold tap or applying an ice pack.

Caution: Be prepared to treat your child for shock after any kind of burn, and keep a careful watch on him. If possible, have someone else take you to the hospital so that you can stay close to your child to comfort him and monitor his breathing. Be prepared and able to administer artificial respiration (*see* **First aid**, page 87) if he becomes unconscious. Do not give him anything to eat or drink. Never put any fats, ointments, lotions or creams onto a burn, break a blister, or cover a burn with a plaster or cotton wool.

Car journeys

Putting your baby into his car seat and going for a drive can be a wonderful way to ease him off to sleep, because the sound of the engine and the movement can be deeply comforting. Just a few years on, however, and the back seat of the car can become a much more troublesome place.

Encourage your children to pay attention to what they can see from their windows by playing 'I spy' and other observation games; keep them occupied with counting and number games or simple geography quizzes. You might want to keep a supply of treats either as prizes or as rewards for good behaviour. A stock of paper and colouring pencils or sticker books can also be useful on particularly long journeys.

Allow a couple of stops on longer journeys for leg-stretching, and so they can burn off excess energy. It's also a good idea to plan around nap times for younger children so that they will sleep for at least part of the journey.

Always keep one window partly open to ensure that there is enough fresh air, and avoid greasy foods and fizzy drinks that may lead to sickness. Encourage children to speak up straight away if they are feeling nauseous or need a toilet stop, and respond to their requests as quickly and as calmly as possible.

See also **Car safety, Travel sickness**

Car safety

All children should be taught from a very early age to remain strapped into their seats at all times. The back doors should have child-proof locks, and seat belts should be installed and checked by a qualified fitter.

The law requires that babies and small children be restrained in a car seat appropriate for their age and weight. There are two main types of seat:

• *Stage 1* – suitable for newborns and babies up to about nine months or 10 kg (22 lbs) in weight. This type of seat can be used in the front seat facing backwards, unless the car has a passenger airbag.

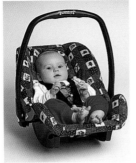

• *Stage 2* – suitable from around nine months and up to about four years or between 9 and 18 kg (20–40 lbs) in weight.

Both types of seat can be bought with special pillows to provide extra comfort. Always ensure that car seats are installed according to instructions or by a qualified fitter.

Note: premature babies and children with special needs may require special arrangements – seek advice from local road safety officers.

> **Caution:** It can be dangerous to leave a baby alone in a stuffy car with the windows shut, even in your own driveway. Always take him out with you even if he is asleep and you don't want to disturb him.

Cardiac massage
See **First aid**

Catarrh

This is an excess of mucus in the nose and throat. It can occur as a symptom of a cold or flu, or it can accompany measles. If your child has an allergy to pollen, catarrh may occur seasonally, as in hay fever, or you may find that it is a reaction to a more common allergen such as dairy foods, or house dust mites' droppings. A build-up of catarrh can lead to sinusitis, coughs, and ear infections.

Teach your child to blow his nose well, from an early age, and check carefully for potential allergens. Reducing dairy products and wheat in the diet may help if the allergy is food-related. Other common allergens include:

- pet hair
- dust (change bedding and freeze toys regularly to kill dust mites)
- chemicals in household cleaners or paints
- cigarette smoke
- air pollution.

Treatment of catarrh depends on the cause. It may simply require removal of the irritant in question or, in the case of hay fever, an antihistamine preparation may be needed. For colds, a steam inhalation can relieve catarrh or a decongestant nose spray from the chemist may help for a few days. A drop of eucalyptus oil or decongestant liquid on your child's pillow could also be helpful.

If symptoms persist for more than four or five days, take your child to the doctor.

> **Caution:** Always consult your doctor if catarrh is making feeding difficult for your baby.

See also **Allergies, Colds**

Check-ups

Your baby's first physical check-up will take place within minutes of his birth. Everything from the number of fingers and toes to his pulse rate and reflexes will be checked by the doctor or midwife.

The APGAR test is so called because it checks **A**ppearance, **P**ulse, **G**rimace, **A**ctivity and **R**espiration. For each part of the test, your baby is given a score of 2 for fully present or fine, 1 for satisfactory, or 0 if there is a problem. An APGAR score of 7, five minutes after birth, is good. A baby scoring less than 4 needs help immediately.

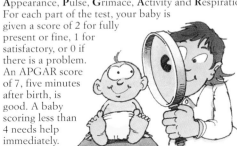

- *Appearance* – if the baby is pink or brown, 2 points; has blue fingers and toes, 1 point; is blue all over 0.
- *Pulse* – over 100, 2 points; under 100, 1 point; not discernible 0.
- *Grimace* or *response to stimulation* – baby cries 2 points; grimaces 1 point; neither 0.
- *Activity* or *muscle tone* – arms and legs move strongly 2 points; are flexed 1 point; floppy 0.
- *Respiration* – strong 2 points; weak and irregular 1 point; absent 0.

At around six to eight weeks, your baby will have a second check-up, again involving a full physical examination including a check on his growth, and you will be offered **vaccinations** for him (*see* page 183). Your baby's growth, size and measurements will be recorded on a chart of standard expected growth curves, and regularly monitored to ensure that he is thriving. The eight-week check is a good opportunity to discuss any queries, worries or uncertainties you may have about your child's progress and care.

At six months you will be offered a hearing test for your child, involving simple distraction techniques. Although fairly crude, this test is a good indicator of any potential hearing problems. The midwife or health visitor will also check your child's eyesight, and whether he is able to sit unsupported, roll over, and play with simple toys such as rattles. You may also be asked questions regarding his responses to strangers and to certain unfamiliar sounds and situations.

At one year babies can have the combined MMR vaccination, then there is a further check-up on their development at about 18 months old. This usually involves asking your child to play with some toys that are specifically designed to assess different areas of his development. He may be watched while he plays to see what he does with the toys and which ones he chooses, or he may be asked to complete specific tasks, such as building a tower with bricks. Results are plotted against charts that show expected limits of development, and the assessor's professional experience will contribute to the findings. This is an opportunity to pick up on any developmental slowness or possible learning disabilities, and if any problems are detected you may be referred to a specialist. If speech is slow, for example, you may be referred to a speech therapist, or it may be suggested that speech development is re-checked at a later date.

Once he goes to school, your child will be looked after by the school welfare officer or nurse, and regular health-checks are required by the education authority.

Chickenpox

This is a common, infectious disease that many children catch. It has an incubation period of about three weeks, and usually causes only mild symptoms. The characteristic itchy spots are sometimes but not always accompanied by a sore throat, headaches and mild fever, but often there is little more than a slight fractiousness or crankiness. The spots can appear anywhere on the body, and quickly develop into tiny blisters that can leave a scar if they are scratched too vigorously. It was once thought that one bout of chickenpox confers lifelong immunity, but there are different strains, and it is possible to get it more than once. The disease is infectious before the first spots appear, until they all have scabs, and your child should be kept away from other people during this period.

Ensure that your child has plenty of rest, and offer a light liquid diet to help him recover. Soothe the itching with regular applications of calamine lotion. Add one drop of lemongrass essential oil to the bath water both to soothe the skin and for its disinfectant qualities, or use an oatmeal pack rather than soap. Keep your child's fingernails short to limit the damage from scratching.

Caution: If spots become further infected, or if your child develops a high fever, headaches or becomes clumsy and disorientated, consult your doctor straight away.

Childminders

Finding someone you are happy to entrust your child to is very important. Informally, this can be a family member or close friend or neighbour, but long-term arrangements tend to be more formal.

It is important to check that the person you choose is registered with the local authority; your nurse or GP should have information about local childminders. Some of the questions you may need to ask are:

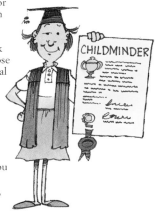

CHILDMINDER

- How flexible can they be over time, e.g. if you need to work late?

- What sort of notice do they need for any changes?

- How long they have been childminding?
- Do they have children of their own?
- How many other children will they be looking after and what ages are they?
- Do they have any helpers?
- Is there an outdoor play area?
- Are there any pets?
- What are their views on discipline?
- What sort of meals/drinks/snacks are offered, and do they cater for special dietary needs?

Ask if you can visit when your childminder is working – this will give you an idea of how happy and occupied the children are. Before you commit, you will want your child to meet the childminder and see how they get along together.

Make sure that the childminder always has contact numbers for you and any back-up friends or family members, and agree the reasons for which you might expect to be called.

Choking

Choking is very serious and can be life-threatening. It occurs when something enters the airway rather than the oesophagus leading to the stomach. With young children this can be anything from a piece of food to a small toy. If there is enough air getting through, they

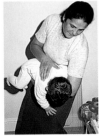

will be able to cough the object back up, but may well need your help.

Lay a baby on your arm or across your lap with his head down and slap him lightly on the back with your other hand. For an older child, picking him up from the waist might be enough to dislodge a particle as you force air up from the diaphragm, before laying him over your lap. If he is able to cough up the article, fish it out of his mouth, taking care not to push it back down again.

Never leave young children to eat unattended, and do not give them nuts or other small pieces of food until they are at least three years old. Teach them that they are not to put small toys into their mouth, and check for small pieces in any toys you give them.

> **Caution:** If your child has difficulty breathing, or you cannot dislodge the article, telephone for an ambulance straight away, or have someone else phone while you continue to try to remove it. For further measures, *see* **First aid**, page 89.

Circumcision

See **Genitals**

Colds

A cold will often leave your child feeling pretty miserable, with any or all of the following symptoms: slight temperature, muscular aches and pains, runny nose, sore throat, cough, catarrh, sneezing and slight headache. In babies and younger children there is also a risk of inner ear infections because the Eustachian tubes are not yet fully grown. Some older children also get earache and may suffer nosebleeds from blowing too hard.

Treat your child with lots of warm drinks. Resist the desire to dose him with small amounts of adult medication. If congestion is a problem and breathing becomes difficult, raise your child's head by putting a pillow under the top of the mattress, and place one drop of eucalyptus oil on his pillow. Keep the air in the room moist (place a bowl of water near the radiator), and smear a little Vaseline or olive oil around your child's nose to prevent soreness. Teach him to blow his nose, and provide lots of treats to make the time pass well.

Caution: Consult your doctor immediately if the infection seems to have travelled to the chest making breathing difficult, or if your baby or child is having difficulty feeding.

See also **Catarrh, Coughs, Earache**

Colic

Many young babies suffer with colic. The characteristic symptoms are:

- crying (often in the early evening), sometimes for hours at a time
- becoming red-faced
- arching his body away from you, or drawing up his knees as if in pain.

It is extremely distressing to see your baby in such obvious discomfort, but colic is totally harmless. Nobody is completely sure what causes it, but it could be some kind of spasm in the gut, or a build-up of gas if he hasn't been winded properly. Taking babies off cow's milk formula, and removing dairy products from the mother's diet if breast-feeding have been known to show good results. Usually it clears up by the time a baby is 12 weeks old.

  If your baby seems to be in pain, rock him, while rubbing his back, and hold him close to you while you walk around. Try sitting him up and burping him, then lay him down on his tummy across your lap. Gripe water or weak dill tea can be effective with some babies. Try giving your baby a warm bath to help him to relax, or apply a warm facecloth to his abdomen.

Comfort behaviours

These can range from head-banging (this may also be attention-seeking), thumb- or dummy-sucking, nail-biting, gentle rocking and genital holding, to wanting to cling on to a favourite toy or blanket (these should be washed now and again). Your child will outgrow them quite naturally, and often the less fuss that is made about them, the less likely they are to become part of everyday behaviour.

A good time to try to wean your child off his comfort behaviour is just before he starts school or nursery. If it involves a toy or blanket, suggest he leaves it behind when you go out and gradually phase it out until he is only using it at night. At the same time, make sure he is feeling secure in other ways; it helps if he has a routine that he likes and can depend upon, and his own special place where he can go to be on his own – this doesn't have to be anywhere large or special, it can simply be his bed, just so long as he knows it is his own safe place. Keep as stable an emotional environment as possible at home so that in time he will learn that security comes from within.

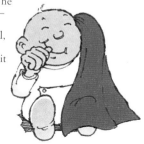

Sometimes comfort behaviours will reappear at times of stress or transition, for example when starting school or moving house. Explain to your child then that there is nothing wrong with using a short-term aid, and that it can be a useful way to feel better in the midst of change. Tell your child's teacher, or other adults who will be responsible for him, about his behaviour, and if it concerns you at all, or is appearing to hold your child back, then discuss the behaviour with your GP or health visitor.

See also **Dummies, Thumb-sucking**

Concussion

See **Head injuries**

Constipation

Constipation, when stools are hard and difficult to pass, is rarely a problem with new babies, but can occur once solid foods are introduced.

Some children have more than one bowel movement a day, while others may go three days before having one, so it is important to know your child's natural rhythm and you need only become concerned when this changes. If your child is basically happy, energetic and otherwise healthy, there is little cause for concern.

If you think your baby is constipated, continue to give him drinks – the best cure is an extra bottle of water a day. Check his tummy for tightness or pain.

Avoid giving laxatives to babies or children. Check your child's stools for any obvious problems, like undigested (and recognizable) pieces of food, or blood.

Make sure that your child's diet includes plenty of liquid, and ample fibre from fruit and vegetables. Ensure that he knows how to respond to the feeling that he needs to go to the toilet and, if he is using a potty or the toilet, check that he feels comfortable using it, and that he has the privacy to do so.

> **Caution:** If there is any pain in the abdomen, or if you discover blood in the stools, contact your GP straight away. Do this too if the constipation does not resolve itself after one week.

Conversation

See **Talking**

Cot death

Cot death is the sudden unexpected death of a baby for no obvious reason. It is the most common cause of death in infants under a year old.

Scientists are still researching the causes of cot death, but it appears there are a number of different factors that can make a baby more vulnerable. While there doesn't seem to be a genetic predisposition, premature babies and those from multiple births are more at risk, and childcare choices also play a part.

The following steps are thought to minimize the risk of cot death:

- Make regular checks on sleeping babies.
- Lay your baby on his back to sleep, not on his side or tummy.
- Choose blankets rather than a duvet, and tuck them in well.
- Place your baby towards the bottom end of the cot so that he cannot slide down under the covers.
- Do not allow your baby to become too hot.
- Do not place the cot near a window or next to a radiator.
- Do not smoke, and do not allow anyone to smoke in the same room as your baby.
- Do not take recreational drugs, and limit your alcohol intake.
- Always buy a new – not second-hand – firm mattress.
- Seek prompt medical advice if your baby is unwell.

Keep your baby in your room at night. A cot that has a side opening allowing it to be placed flush with your own bed is a good idea. You might also consider using a baby alarm that will alert you if the baby's breathing stops or if the temperature rises or falls outside an optimum range.

Coughs

A cough is an automatic reaction as your body tries to clear the throat of some irritation or blockage. It can be the sign of an illness, like a cold, or something more serious such as asthma or whooping cough. Coughing accompanied by pain may be an indication of a more serious condition, such as pleurisy. Coughs will also occur in a smoke-filled or polluted atmosphere, and can be the result of an allergy.

Soothe your child with plenty of drinks and lots of hot water, lemon and honey. Help him to cough up any phlegm by supporting him as he sits up, and gently rubbing or patting him lightly on the back between the shoulder blades. Check the mucus he coughs up for signs of infection – clear is best, and thick green or blue, or blood-stained, mean you should call the doctor. Prop your child up at night with extra pillows underneath the mattress to make breathing easier, and keep the air in the room clear (open a window) and moist (boil a kettle – out of your child's reach) until breathing is relieved. Ensure that his diet provides adequate vitamin C, and check for potential allergies. Encourage good oral hygiene, and if your child is old enough, a light salt mouthwash will keep bacteria at bay, stopping one avenue of infection.

If your child is repeatedly ill with a cough, or if it lasts for more than two days, consult your doctor.

Caution: If symptoms worsen, if breathing becomes difficult, or if coughing is accompanied by pain or blood, seek urgent medical attention.

Cradle cap

This is a covering of thick, greasy scaling on the scalp that sometimes extends over the face and behind the ears and down the neck as well. It is quite common in babies and can last for some time. Cradle cap is greasy to the touch, and causes flaking of the skin but, although unpleasant to look at, it does not usually cause your baby much irritation. It is a form of dermatitis, and will usually disappear of its own accord.

Continue to shampoo your baby's hair with a mild baby shampoo, but if the condition persists treat with regular applications of small amounts of baby oil or warmed olive oil, rubbing it in gently all over the affected region. Use a very soft bristle brush to brush away loose flakes between oil treatments. Symptoms

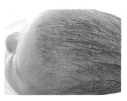

can recur, and will respond to the same treatment. Some experts think that cradle cap is related to a fungal infection, so extra care should be taken over hygiene to protect against recurrence. Apply calendula cream to the area if the baby is troubled by the condition, and if any scabbing or bleeding occurs, consult your GP straight away. If you notice similar patches elsewhere on your baby's body, it may be a sign of eczema or another skin complaint requiring proper diagnosis.

See also **Eczema**

Crawling

Most babies usually start crawling between six months and one year, often going backwards at first. This is the first time they will be able to move around with any real independence, and is an important building block in their self-esteem. There are some children who simply don't do it, however, moving straight into standing and tottering around, while others move predominantly sideways, or might shuffle along on their bottoms.

Once your child begins to crawl, you will need to

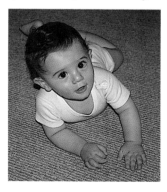

make sure that his world is a safe place for him. It is a good idea to sit on the floor at his level, and have a look around for danger points. Cover or protect sharp edges on tables and other furniture, remove possible climbing aids like low drawer handles, and ensure that all electric cables and sockets are covered. Remove tablecloths and other loose pieces of fabric that can be pulled down by your baby.

Once your baby is mobile, his natural curiosity will lead him to explore. If he spots something of interest, he will be able to cover seemingly large distances very quickly so it's particularly important that he is not left unattended.

Croup

This is a cough that sounds dry and 'barking', and occurs in very young children whose underdeveloped bronchial tubes can easily become constricted or blocked with mucus. It often occurs after a cold or infection such as bronchitis, but it can also be a symptom of an allergy.

The onset of croup is usually very quick, often during the night, and coughing may last for a couple of hours. You may also notice a slightly raised temperature and the child will be restless.

Sit your child up to help him to breathe, either propping him up with pillows or taking him on to your lap. Remember that breathing-related difficulties can be very scary so reassure him. Moist air will help, so boil a kettle (out of his reach) in the room, or sit him on your lap in the bathroom for a while with the hot water tap running so that he can inhale the steam. Open a window in his bedroom if the weather is damp, but protect against draughts. Central heating tends to dry the air so either turn it off in his room, or place a bowl of water by the radiator. Humidifiers can also be a good investment.

Caution: If your child's breathing becomes laboured or you notice any blueness around his face and mouth, contact the emergency services right away.

Crying

Your baby's cry is his way of communicating with you in the early months before other skills and forms of communication have developed. All babies cry, and some cry more than others. You will soon be able to distinguish whether your baby is crying because he wants comfort, because he is anxious, lonely or fearful, or because he is hungry. Some babies will also cry to tell you that their nappy is full. If your baby is crying, pick him up and offer a

feed, or if you have recently fed him, just offer some
cooled boiled water. Check that his nappy is clean, and
that he is not too hot or too cold. It may simply be that
he wants to be near you.

Continuous crying may be a sign of some physical
concern, and it is important to consult your doctor.

A crying baby can place an enormous strain on the
mother or primary carer. Always seek help and support
for yourself if you find your baby too demanding.

If your baby or young child is very dependent on
you, and cries when you are not around, consider
carrying him with you in a baby sling or settle him in a
bouncing chair within full view of you. This may be
enough to reassure him and stop the crying.

If your child is over six months old and is still crying,
and you have ruled out causes such as teething, colic
and physical discomfort, try providing him with as
many sources of stimulation as possible – it may simply
be that he is bored. It is also a good idea to review
feeding habits, and check for possible allergies to dairy
products that could be causing problems.

See also **Colic**

Cuts

Once your child is walking or crawling, he is going to
pick up simple cuts and grazes, bumps and bruises, no
matter how hard you try to protect him. Any injury to
the skin that damages the tissue and causes bleeding

needs to be treated. Always wash with salty water, or use a mild antiseptic. Pat the skin dry very gently and if the cut is in an exposed spot requiring extra protection, like a knee, cover it with a plaster. There will often also be bruising underneath and around the cut.

If the cut looks deep or if bleeding will not stop, you must get medical help straight away. Get a clean cloth or bandage, hold it firmly on to the site of the bleeding, and hold that part up in the air above the level of his heart. This will slow down the blood flow. Lay your child down and keep him warm and comforted until help arrives. Even if the bleeding stops in response to your treatment, you should seek medical care in case of shock or any infection setting in. The wound may also need to be stitched closed.

See also **Bruises**

Diarrhoea

This is the frequent passing of loose, watery stools and it can seriously dehydrate babies and young children.

The most common causes of diarrhoea are infections or irritation in the gut, and these can be caused by food allergy or by viruses or bacteria in foods. Personal hygiene is essential in minimizing the contamination of food; always wash your hands before preparing food, before and after changing your baby's nappy, after using the toilet and after gardening or doing outside work. Encourage older children to do the same. Sterilize all babies' feeding equipment (*see* page 33), and don't allow anyone who has diahorrea to be in contact with your baby.

If your baby gets diarrhoea, continue to feed him as usual, and supplement feeds with bottles of cooled boiled water. Older children can be given drinks of diluted fruit juice, or water to which you have added a pinch of salt and a teaspoon of sugar. Keep your child warm and comfortable, and check his temperature. If it is raised, cool him down with tepid sponging, but do not allow him to become chilled.

Caution: Call your doctor immediately if your child's stools contain mucus or blood, if diarrhoea is accompanied by vomiting or abdominal pain, or if symptoms persist for more than six hours.

See also **Drinking liquids**

Disability

Parents of children born with an obvious disability will have access to a great deal of professional support and they will receive advice on any special training or equipment that their child will need. However, minor physical and mental disabilities are often accepted by a loving family, and it is only when the child begins to mix with others that difficulties and even prejudice can cause problems. Try to equip your child as far as possible to face such challenges, and be prepared yourself for awkward encounters. Often people simply do not know what to say or do, but if you can state exactly what additional care or support your child needs, it will make things a lot easier.

Some conditions that can disable your child include deafness and sight loss. These are rare, however, and regular developmental check-ups will catch any early signs or symptoms so be sure to keep your clinic appointments and assessments.

If you notice anything strange in your child's development, or anything that causes you concern, discuss the matter straight away with your doctor.

Discipline

Teaching your child personal discipline and behavioural boundaries will help him to handle his feelings more easily, to achieve his aims, and to communicate more effectively in relationships.

Setting strong boundaries within the home gives your child a sense of security – it is natural for him to want to

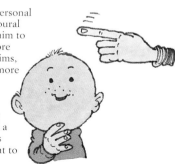

test the limits of new situations, and each time you stand by your word and keep to your routines, you strengthen his sense of acceptable boundaries, and give him confidence. This is especially important within an extended family, where it can be all too easy for a child to go from one adult to another and get a different response. It is crucial for parents and other carers to back each other up over disciplinary issues if the message is to get through.

Decide the rules you think it is most important for your child to adhere to and teach them in a clear, consistent way. These may include a personal hygiene routine, going to bed at specific times, saying 'please' and 'thank you' or, for older children, helping around the house.

If your child misbehaves, you will need to employ a range of strategies to help him learn just what is acceptable. Be clear about what these are, and be sure to stick to your decisions about them – children are very quick to pick up on inconsistencies, particularly those in response to their crying or tantrums. If you threaten to withdraw treats, make sure that you keep to your word. It helps if your punishments are specific and immediate. Incentives also work well, because children will want to please you, so offering treats as rewards for good behaviour will often be more effective than threats about bad behaviour.

See also **Smacking**

Dressing babies and children

Young babies are not very good at regulating their temperature, so keep checking them for temperature changes, and as a general rule dress them in one layer more than you are wearing. For indoor wear, it is important to keep your baby comfortable, warm and protected.

Outdoors, a hat is important to protect from the sun as well as the rain and colder weather (but always remove this indoors). Make sure your baby's pram or pushchair has a screen that will shield him from the

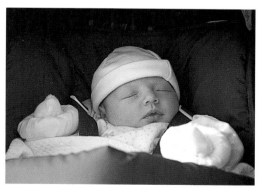

weather, and always carry an extra layer with you in case the weather becomes cooler.

It is more difficult to keep toddlers and older children well wrapped up. They may want to tear jackets off to give them extra mobility. High levels of activity will help them keep warm at the time, but it is vital that you add an extra layer immediately afterwards, when they will be prone to chilling. Layers of light clothing that can easily be added to and removed are the best choice.

For babies, clothes that open down the front or with wide envelope necks are always best. Also look out for clothes that do not have to be completely removed for nappy changing, and those with wide sleeves rather than tiny armholes to battle with. Dress your baby on a flat surface and guide his head and arms gently through openings so that his nose and fingers don't get squashed or caught.

When dressing young children, take care not to bend malleable arms and legs too much, and make getting dressed and undressed into a fun thing to do together. Encourage children to play a part in their own dressing – choosing between two suitable options, or picking the colour they want to wear should help to eliminate any conflict. Introduce them to dexterity skills like doing up buttons and tying bows in shoelaces as soon as their fingers can manage.

See also **Sunburn**

Drinking liquids

Dehydration is a concern when children are unwell, have a fever, or are vomiting or have diarrhoea. In babies you will notice that the **fontanelle** (*see* page 93) becomes sunken, and their urine becomes concentrated and darker in colour. This can occur quite easily, especially when weaning, because both breast- and formula milk have a high percentage of water, and when they are replaced by solid food, your child's fluid level may be reduced without your even realizing. Make sure you give plenty of drinks, and if you notice dehydration, or even dry mouth and lips and lethargy, then give small amounts every ten minutes or so. Choose water or diluted fruit juices.

Babies and young children are prone to putting things in their mouths and then they will naturally swallow. Curiosity may lead them to sample water from flower vases and from toilets or drains, so take great care when adding cleaning fluids or flower preservatives and other chemicals.

Around the house, cleaning fluids and bleaches under the sink will need to be locked away, as will disinfectants and toilet cleaners. You will also need to protect your children from drinking alcohol, perfume, cosmetics and pharmaceuticals. As children get older, simply placing items out of reach may not be enough of a safeguard. Although it is a chore, locking liquids and other dangerous substances away is the only sure way to guarantee your child's safety.

> **Caution:** If your child does drink something he shouldn't, ring the emergency services or take him to the nearest hospital straight away. Always take the bottle or a sample of whatever he has drunk with you if possible.

See also **First aid, Safety**

Drowning

Young children can drown in only 5 cm (2 in) of water or other fluid, so it is essential that they are not left unattended in the bath, or near open water. Safeguarding your home and garden and adopting good practices will dramatically reduce the risk:

- Never let your child out of your sight when you are near water – even a paddling pool.

- Make sure that your child learns to swim as early as possible.

- Warn your child of the dangers that water can pose as soon as he is old enough to understand.

- Never let your child swim out to sea after a stray beach ball or float in the sea on an air-mattress.

- Take note of any warning flags on beaches.

- Do not allow children to swim after a heavy meal.

If your child is drowning, you will need to act quickly. Young children have an instinctive ability to survive for longer than you would think when underwater and cold, so do not give up on any life-saving measure, but keep it going until help arrives.

Remove your child from the water as quickly and easily as you can. If you can hook him out using an arm, a pole or a life belt, this is better than diving in after him. If your child is conscious, take him somewhere warm, and change him into fresh dry clothes. If he is unconscious, give mouth-to-mouth resuscitation (*see* **First aid**) immediately and keep going until breathing starts or medical help arrives. Once breathing starts, cover your child with whatever layers you have available to keep him warm, and stay close to him. In all cases you will need to go to the nearest casualty department as quickly as possible. If you have to drive there, keep a constant check on your child to make sure that he is breathing, and be prepared to stop and administer mouth-to-mouth resuscitation again if he should stop.

Most children will recover from incidents like this without any ongoing problems, but it is essential that they receive a medical check-up in even minor cases.

Dummies

It is an undisputed fact that many babies are soothed by sucking on something. For many people a dummy

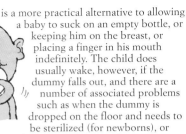

is a more practical alternative to allowing a baby to suck on an empty bottle, or keeping him on the breast, or placing a finger in his mouth indefinitely. The child does usually wake, however, if the dummy falls out, and there are a number of associated problems such as when the dummy is dropped on the floor and needs to be sterilized (for newborns), or when it is lost and a new one is rejected.

Buying a good supply of dummies once you have found one your baby likes is a good idea. It is also worth considering an orthodontic dummy if your baby gets on with it as these are thought to be better for gums and teeth.

Usually by the time the child is 2–3 years old he becomes less reliant on the dummy, and may be able to do without it for longer periods. This is a good opportunity to suggest he might like to give it up, or even give it away. Otherwise, before he starts nursery or school, you should start to encourage him to leave it behind, gradually phasing it out, so that he only uses it at night, and eventually not at all.

Caution: Never soak your baby's dummy in anything like sugar, alcohol, fruit juice or honey.

See also **Comfort behaviours, Thumb sucking**

Earache

Ear infections are very common in babies and young children, and will often be caused by a viral or bacterial infection in the throat or nose. They tend to come on quite quickly, often at night or when lying down because this increases pressure in the ear.

You would suspect an ear infection if your child is:

• irritable and clingy

• running a temperature, or feverish

• suffering with cold-type symptoms

• crying, particularly when lying down

• pulling at his ear or favouring one side of the head

• red around the ear, or has a discharge from the ear.

Treatment at home can include wrapping a warm hot water bottle in a soft towel, and holding it against his ear. Calpol (a paracetamol preparation) can be given to babies over three months old to soothe the pain. Any discharge from the ear can be wiped away gently with a clean flannel dipped in warm water. Keep him upright, and don't prod or poke around the ear. Keep the area dry and warm, and away from wind or draughts.

Your child should be taken to the GP with any type of ear infection as a course of antibiotics may be required.

> **Caution:** Have your child's ears checked within two weeks of any ear infection to confirm that they are clear and to check that no damage has been done.

See also **Glue ear**

Eating problems

Being relaxed at mealtimes or during feeds, and introducing your child slowly, carefully, and as early as possible to a wide range of foods will go a long way towards preventing eating problems.

Babies often know best what suits them and what doesn't, so if they continually reject a certain food, accept that and seek alternatives. Young children can become a bit faddy about foods, eating some for a period of time, and then changing their favourites and their dislikes, seemingly on a whim. Provided their diet is not becoming too limited nutritionally (for example, consisting solely of peanut butter), calmly indulge them. There will also be periods when they natur-ally don't

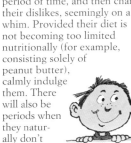

feel hungry and don't want to eat. Don't let refusal to eat become a weapon. Take food away if it's not eaten and don't fill him up with sweet things. A hungry child is less likely to refuse food at the next meal. Keep your cool.

Introduce your children, especially girls, to good eating habits from their first meals (this is because there is a higher incidence of eating disorders among growing girls than boys). Encourage a calm atmosphere and respect for food and each other. Avoid over-reliance on any one type of food, and do not keep condiments like salt and pepper on the table. Fads and fussy eating can be dealt with more easily if good dietary basics have been established early on.

See also **Mealtimes, Nutrition**

The following tips may help if mealtimes are threatening to become difficult:

- Try not to get angry, and avoid confrontations.

- Be positive – offer an incentive rather than threatening: 'after your main course you can have some jelly', and not 'there'll be no jelly if you don't have your main course'.

- Don't impose rules that you don't have the time or patience to enforce.

- Always make your child sit at the table at mealtimes – eventually, he will probably want to join in.

Eczema

One in eight children suffers from eczema at some point, although 70 per cent will outgrow it by their teens. This irritating condition in which the skin becomes dry, scaly and itchy, and sometimes forms blisters, can appear anywhere on the body, but common sites include the face, hands, armpits and inner elbows, behind the knees, and the groin. Causes include allergies, and the incidence of eczema is highest in families where there are other allergies.

Eczema will often appear for the first time when solids are introduced into your child's diet. Keeping dairy products and wheat out of the diet will help to reduce the problem, as will minimizing contact with other possible allergens such as pets, lanolin, biological detergents and synthetic fabrics.

Treat by moisturizing the skin regularly, having oatmeal baths, and keeping cool. Your doctor may prescribe an emollient cream such as E45, which can either be applied direct to affected areas, or used in the bath. Sometimes a steroid cream is prescribed for short-term use.

Choose cotton bedding and clothing, and keep your child's nails short so that scratching does not break the skin. Treat the house regularly for house dust mites (put cuddly toys in a plastic bag and freeze overnight at least once a month).

See also **Allergies, Cradle Cap**

> **Caution:** Do not remove any major foods or food groups from your child's diet without professional advice and monitoring.

E numbers

These are codes identifying substances such as chemical preservatives which are added to foods to enhance their shelf-life, or otherwise change their flavour or colour. Some of the chemicals used in food preparation have been shown to cause allergies and hyperactivity in children.

As a general rule, you should feed your baby on foods that are as natural as possible. Avoid chemical additives and read all labels on food packaging carefully. A good guide is that if the additive doesn't have a name, only a number, it is best to put the product back on the shelf until you can find out more, and choose a product that contains just natural or recognizable ingredients. Fresh, unprocessed and wholesome foods are undoubtedly preferable. Watch out for pre-packaged foods intended for adults, which may contain levels of chemical additives that are dangerous for children.

Eyesight

Your child's eyesight will be checked as part of his physical examinations when he is growing up, but if you have any specific concerns, take him directly to your doctor or to an ophthalmologist.

Your child's eyesight will change in its acuity from a baby's first vision which tends to be hazy and focused on bright or contrasting colours within a specific range, to the good general eyesight that can be expected from an older child. If your child's attention wanders, or if he is slow in picking up skills like reading, it may be time to have his eyes checked.

We exercise our eyes naturally when changing focus and looking at an object that is close by and then at one further away. Children do this instinctively as part of their inquisitiveness and joy in discovering the world, but there may be times when you need to discourage bad habits like long stretches of sitting and watching TV.

Teach your child not to rub his eyes, and always to take great care not to poke himself or put dirty fingers near his eyes. If something does enter the eye, have your child blow his nose – this sometimes clears it. If not, gently open the eye yourself and see if you can fish it out with the tip of a cotton handkerchief, or pull the upper lid down over the lower lid once or twice. Holding the eye open for a moment will often allow it to naturally produce tears and cleanse itself.

> **Caution:** If any foreign object enters the eye and is not easily removed, take your child immediately to the nearest surgery or hospital.

Falls

Tumbles and falls will often happen as your child explores and encounters the world around him and gains confidence and co-ordination. Once walking is mastered, scraped hands and knees are inevitable and it is important for your child's confidence that you are not over-protective of him, while at the same time ensuring that he is safe. Any anxiety will be picked up by him, and will only inhibit him. Allow him to pick himself up after a tumble.

Most injuries will be nothing more than a minor irritation. If your child is often falling off things, it is worth checking his upper body strength as well as his ability to concentrate on the task in hand. Your district nurse or GP will be able to help you with this. Otherwise, check for common causes such as undone shoelaces, forgetting about a step, or general lack of co-ordination. Often the cause is likely to be sheer impatience and an overdose of enthusiasm on your child's part.

Caution:

- If your child seems to be constantly falling over, have his gait and co-ordination checked by your GP or a paediatrician.
- If he has fallen and there is bad bruising, serious bleeding or concussion take him to the hospital straight away.
- Seek medical advice if your child is still complaining of pain some hours after a blow to the head even if there is no visible sign of injury.

See also **Cuts, Bruises, Fractures**

Fears

Children can become frightened by any number of real or imagined things. Babies and toddlers may become startled by loud noises or sudden jerky movements. With older children, causes can include separation anxiety, being bullied at school, discipline at home enforced through fear, or just over-active imaginations. Fears can manifest in bedwetting, headaches, nightmares and disruptive behaviour, as well as through tantrums and tears. It is important to take a child's fears seriously, and not to belittle them, but use gentle teasing and reassurance to restore his confidence.

Information usually helps to dispel fears, so encourage your child to follow his natural curiosity and learn about any specific causes of anxiety, e.g. spiders. Simple practical strategies can also be very helpful – leaving a hall light on to alleviate fears of the dark, etc. Also, try not to show your own feelings of fear in a frightening situation, but react calmly to set an example.

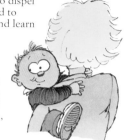

See also **Bullying, Separation anxiety**

Fever

Your child's normal body temperature is 36–37° C (96.8–98° F). A temperature of over 37.7° C (100° F) is potentially serious if your baby is less than six months old and medical help should be sought. Read a baby's temperature by putting a thermometer under his armpit, or using a forehead sticker with a digital read-out. You can buy these at any chemist. You can sometimes tell by simply placing your hand on his forehead, and seeing if it feels hot and dry or clammy.

Children will tend to have a raised temperature when they are teething, or if they are over-excited or have been running around energetically. A fever can also be a symptom of a bacterial or viral infection. If your child is unwell, and his raised temperature lasts for more than a few hours, or is not completely relieved by any measures you take, then consult your GP.

If your child has a fever, loosen any tight clothing, place damp towels on his forehead, sponge him down with tepid water, and give only liquids to drink, no food.

> **Caution:** Fever is one symptom of **meningitis** (*see* page 127), a life-threatening concern. If your child has a fever, especially with cold hands or feet, and you have a sense that something is wrong, contact your GP immediately.

See also **Temperature**

Fever fits

Fever fits, or febrile convulsions, are violent, involuntary movements of the body. These are experienced by around 1 in 20 children and can be very frightening for the parent. The most common cause of convulsions is a high body temperature. If other members of the family have suffered from fever fits, your child is more likely to have them, but will usually grow out of them by the age of about five.

The fits may start with the child becoming unconscious. He may then twitch and writhe, clench his teeth, froth at the mouth, and empty his bowels and bladder. A few minutes later he may briefly become conscious again and then fall asleep.

Stay with your child during the convulsions. Lay him on his front, so that if he vomits, there is no danger of him choking. If you can put a clean pad between his teeth it will prevent him from biting his tongue. Do not restrain him, but protect him from striking his head on any objects. When he is still, place him in the recovery position (*see* **First aid**) and contact your GP. Stay with your child all the time. Try to cool his fever by wrapping a damp cloth around his head. If your child is prone to fever fits, keeping him cool when he has a temperature by bathing him with tepid water, may prevent them.

See also **Fever, Temperature**

Fighting

Children can sometimes fight quite nastily, but this is often easily remedied. It is important to find out why they are fighting, but your initial action must always be to separate them. It is very important that the children do not actually hurt each other, and once apart it will be easier for them to settle down. It is not always easy to part warring children, but younger children can often be simply disentangled. Older infants may need to be sent to opposite ends of the room, or even placed in separate rooms till they are calm.

All the children involved need to be heard before they will be ready to begin to understand each other, and move towards 'making up'. If you can speak to them separately first, and then bring them together to discuss what has happened, the resolution should be speedy. Younger children may simply need to have it clearly explained to them that this sort of behaviour is unacceptable.

Very young children can't be reasoned with – if they are biting or hitting you will have to remove them from the situation immediately. Try to encourage them to express their aggression in other ways such as banging a drum or punching a cushion.

Children can become aggressive for any number of background reasons, such as sibling rivalry, or upsets in the home. If your child is continually troubled, and taking it out on others, do involve their play-school worker, and any other adults that care for them, in resolving their behaviour.

Punishing other people's children (whether physically or otherwise) is not generally acceptable, but if there is a disturbance that you cannot contain, contact the child's parents to have them taken home or away from you, and supervise the children until this happens.

See also **Bullying, Discipline, Sibling rivalry**

First aid

You will almost certainly have to cope with some accidents while your child is young. It is likely that most of them will be minor, but you should be prepared for a major accident. Ideally, you should go on a first aid course, but if this is not possible, then buy a good book and make sure that you are familiar with the most essential points. It is also important to have a first aid kit in the house, where you can get at it easily, but where it is out of the reach of children.

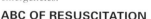

This section gives some of the first aid essentials for use in emergencies.

ABC OF RESUSCITATION

If you find your child lying on the floor and think that he has stopped breathing, first check that the cause is not something that will put you in danger, such as contact with a live wire. If you are sure that it is safe to approach, try gently shaking him or pinching him. Call his name and if there is still no response, immediately call for help and then follow the ABC of resuscitation as follows:

A – open the airway
1 Place your child on a firm surface.
2 Look in his mouth for any obstruction which can be removed easily.
3 Put your hand on his forehead and gently lift his chin with two fingers. DO NOT touch the back of his throat as this may cause the palate to swell and further block the airway.

B – check breathing
1 Put your ear close to your child's mouth.
2 Look to see if the chest is rising and falling.
3 Listen for sounds of breathing.
4 Feel for breath on your cheek.
If your child is not breathing begin artificial respiration (see opposite).

C – check circulation
For babies: check the pulse inside the upper arm by lightly pressing two fingers towards the bone.
For children: check the pulse in the neck by lightly pressing two fingers to one side of the windpipe.

Note: If your child has a pulse but is not breathing start artificial respiration (*see* opposite). If he has no pulse after five seconds start chest compression (*see* page 88) together with artificial respiration.

If he has a pulse and is breathing place him in the recovery position (*see* page 89) and dial 999. Continue to check breathing and pulse frequently.

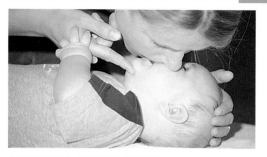

ARTIFICIAL RESPIRATION

For babies (up to 12 months)
1 Seal your lips around his mouth and nose.
2 Blow gently, looking along his chest as you breathe.
3 As the chest rises, stop blowing and allow it to fall.
4 Do this at a rate of 20 breaths per minute until the chest begins to rise by itself.

For children (over 12 months)
1 Seal your lips around the child's mouth, while pinching his nose.
2 Blow gently, looking along his chest as you breathe. Take shallow breaths and do not empty your lungs completely.
3 As the chest rises, stop blowing and allow it to fall.
4 Do this at a rate of 20 breaths per minute until the chest begins to rise by itself.

CHEST COMPRESSION

This should always be combined with artificial
respiration.

For babies (up to 12 months)
1 Place your baby on a firm surface.
2 Find the correct position – a finger's width below the
nipple line, in the middle of the chest.
3 Press two fingers down on the chest by 2 cm (1 in).
4 Press five times in about three seconds then blow
once gently into the lungs.
5 Continue for one minute.
6 Take your baby with you to a phone and call 999.
7 Continue resuscitation until help arrives.

For children (over 12 months)
1 Place one hand two fingers' width above the edge
where the ribs meet the breastbone.
2 Use the heel of that hand to press down by 3 cm.
3 Press five times in about three seconds then blow
once gently into the lungs.
4 Continue for one minute.
5 Take your child with you to a phone and call 999.
6 Continue resuscitation until help arrives.

RECOVERY POSITION.

For babies (up to 12 months)
Do not use the recovery position. Hold your baby face
down in your arms with his head kept low.

For children (over 12 months)
1 Place the arm nearest to you at right angles to the
body, elbow bent. Bring the other arm across the
chest. Hold the hand, palm out, against the cheek.
2 Roll your child on to his side so the upper leg is bent
at the knee and arms remain as above.
3 Tilt his head back gently to keep the airway open.

HEIMLICH MANOEUVRE

If your child is choking and you are unable to shift the
blockage in his airway, you will have to carry out the
Heimlich manoeuvre. Place yourself behind your child
and steady him with one arm. Put your other arm
around him and position the heel of your hand on his
upper abdomen. Give a sharp pull upwards and
inwards below his ribs. Repeat up to five times. If this
does not work and you have not already called an
ambulance, call it now and continue repeating a
sequence of back slaps and abdominal thrusts. If your
child becomes unconscious, follow the ABC of
resuscitation (*see page 86*).

BROKEN BONES

If the bone is bent or curved or sticking through the
skin, call an ambulance. Do not move your child
unless you have to. Drape a sterile dressing over the
site of any wound but do not apply pressure and do
not try to clean or touch the wound.

   If your child cannot move that body part but there is
no obvious bone sticking through the skin, immobilize

the area by taping or wrapping the joints above and below the injury, and take him to hospital. Do not give him anything to eat or drink. Keep him warm and as calm as possible.

See also specific entries under **Burns, Choking, Cuts, Drowning, Fractures, Head injuries, Stings**

First foods

Wait until your baby is at least four months old before introducing solids. Some children do not begin until they are six months old.

When you first introduce foods, make sure that they are liquidized and easy to take, keeping them close to the consistency of milk, and giving only small amounts. Start with a taste on the tip of your finger or a rounded plastic spoon and slowly increase the amount. Always wait at least a couple of days between starting one new food and the next so that it will be easier to pinpoint the source if there are any allergic reactions.

Start giving 'solids' at just one feed per day, and after a few weeks introduce them at a second feed, increasing the amount to 1–2 teaspoonsful. There is no rush. By the end of a six- to eight-week period your baby should be eating solids three times a day – at breakfast, lunch and dinner time – and by the time he is one year old he will be able to have three meals and two snacks a day.

In the early stages it is worth preparing vegetables and freezing them in ice cube trays so that you have the right amount for each meal, rather than preparing a tiny bit each time. Take care when reheating foods in the microwave, stirring well to remove 'hot spots'.

For first foods consider:

• baby rice
• mashed potato
• mashed banana
• puréed fruit, e.g. apple, pear, apricot
• puréed vegetables, e.g. carrot, courgette.

Once your baby is coping well with these, you can start to thicken them, making them lumpier and less runny as he starts to get some teeth. He should be able to eat mashed rather than puréed foods by the time he is about eight months, and this is a good introduction to chewing. Towards one year of age, you can start to include finely chopped foods, and a wider variety of meals, adding pulses and other proteins.

The foods and tastes you are introducing your baby to now may influence his palate for the rest of his life. Do not season his food with salt and pepper, or add sugar and other sweeteners, and do not be tempted to include chillies and other strong spices. Wait as long as you can (never younger than six months, better if he is one year old) before introducing wheat and wheat products, nuts and nut products, fried or fatty foods, dairy products like yoghurt, cheese and fromage frais (unless modified for babies), eggs and citrus fruits.

Commercial baby foods are useful but should not replace home-made foods altogether. Always check that seals on cans and jars have not been broken and look carefully at the labels, making sure that foods are suitable for your baby's age and stage of weaning and that they contain no added sugar or sweeteners and minimal salt. There is a wide range of meals and snacks on the market including many organic choices.

Your baby will probably want to feed himself, but eating with his hands will be his chosen method until he is around two years old. Encourage this with finger-friendly foods like lightly steamed carrots and florets of broccoli; cut fruits, bread and pieces of chicken into easily-held fingers. Some mothers find finger foods help to distract a child, allowing you to spoon puréed foods into his mouth without a fuss.

Make sure you observe good food hygiene from the start, and encourage your child to wash his hands before and after meals. Do not force your child if he is not hungry. Children naturally have periods when they do not feel like eating. Trust their judgement, so long as they do not continue without feeding for more than a day, but make sure they drink plenty of liquids.

See also **Eating problems, Nutrition, Weaning**

Fontanelles

These are soft spots on a baby's head where the bones of the skull have not yet formed or fused. The largest of these – the anterior (front) fontanelle – is on the top of the baby's head; it is diamond-shaped and measures approximately 4 cm (1½ inches) across. Fontanelles provide the potential space for the baby's head to contract as he passes through the birth canal. It takes a while for the bones of the skull to grow and for that area to harden, and until then the fontanelles will be covered by a strong, protective membrane.

Caution: If the fontanelle ever looks swollen, or sunken, or otherwise changed, consult your doctor straight away because this can be an indication of an immediate health concern.

Fractures

Fractures are broken bones. Young children's bones are supple and they can fracture relatively easily, and without the symptoms that could be expected in adults. Their bones often 'crack' rather than break completely and these fractures are known as 'hairline' or greenstick fractures.

If you suspect that your child has hurt himself, perhaps as the result of a fall or knock, then make sure that he is seen by your GP or take him to the hospital. An x-ray is often the only way to tell for sure if your child has a fracture or a broken bone, and this can be done easily and safely while you are present. Unless your child is in a lot of pain, having an x-ray taken can be made into something of a game, and being able to see the 'photo' afterwards is often a big treat and can earn him lots of 'street cred' if he can take a copy to show his friends.

Treatment will depend on the site of the fracture and may be nothing more than binding. If the injury needs plaster, you will need to keep it dry, and help your child to remain as active as possible in spite of it. Most breaks heal in six to ten weeks; in babies they can heal in as little as two weeks. Your doctor will advise if any exercise or physiotherapy is needed.

See **First aid,** page 89

Friendships

Encourage your child to make friends among his peers. Children learn through their relationships, and their future socialization will be influenced by early experiences. Through friendship your child will learn about give and take, sharing and the boundaries of acceptable behaviour. It also gives him scope to build on his ability to relate, and develop a range of other skills such as conversation.

Mother and toddler groups are a good way to encourage early friendships for your child. In early years, children will play alongside one another without seeming to interact, but gradually they will learn to play 'together'. Children form their first real friendships around the age of three or four, but those with older siblings may well have better social skills and be better at adapting, so they will form relationships earlier. Encourage them to share their toys, and support these early friendships as much as possible, perhaps by inviting other children round to play at your house for the afternoon.

It is important to supervise children while they play together, and to provide a structure for the friendships. Be prepared to arrange sleepovers, trips out and shared mealtimes as the children grow older and friendships begin to develop, but always check with other children's parents that arrangements suit them as well.

Friendships with much older children or young adults should be carefully monitored and viewed with caution. Make sure that you feel entirely confident that older friends are trustworthy and reliable.

Imaginary friends can be great playmates and companions for your child. Do not discourage them, and allow your child to include them in his fantasy world, incorporating them into the different games and scenarios that he may invent. Sometimes these friends are secret, but often your child would like them to be included in the family, so try to show interest in them, and check where they are (so as not to sit on them) and what they want to do. These friends can be a useful voice for a child who lacks the confidence to say and do certain things himself. Imaginary friends usually 'go away' by the time your child is of school age.

See also **Sibling rivalry**

Genitals

Your baby will receive a thorough physical check-up shortly after birth to ensure that he is completely well and that there are no obvious abnormalities. A baby's genitals look very much like those of an adult, except in size and colouring. Sometimes, especially in premature babies, the testicles have not descended at birth but they should do so over the next few months.

Always be very gentle when cleaning around the genital area. Do not be surprised if it provokes urination, particularly when cleaning around a boy's foreskin. No attempt should be made to pull back a boy's foreskin or the lips of a girl's vulva for cleaning or for any other reason.

Circumcision – removal of the foreskin – is carried out for cultural or (infrequently) medical reasons, and is best done as soon as possible after the birth.

Older children will need to be encouraged to wash their hands before and after using the toilet, and this is a good time to introduce them to this part of their body, and explain why some degree of privacy is usually employed when involving it.

All children 'explore' their bodies, and if they do not learn shame or anxiety when they begin to do this, they are more likely to grow up free of any hang-ups about their bodies. Children should never be scolded for masturbating, and simple distraction techniques are the best way of dealing with it if they begin to rub themselves in public.

Gifted children

Some children show striking ability in a particular area – perhaps in music, or art, language skills, physical expression or academic achievement. It is important to have any suspected gifts confirmed by a teacher or other professional with experience in working with children, and then it will be easier to obtain the additional support needed.

Children who show academic excellence can have a difficult time in the formal education system. There is nothing worse than letting a child become bored in the classroom because he has already covered the subject being taught. Work closely with your child's teacher or play-leader, and be prepared to consider a range of educational options to ensure that your child is encouraged appropriately and gets the opportunity to flourish.

Individual tuition in an area in which he excels and/or the development of some other skill outside school, such as chess or dance or another language, for as long as he enjoys it, is a good starting point. Make sure you encourage his efforts and results, but always

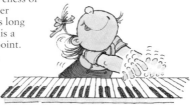

reinforce the fact that it is the child you love, not his achievements, and don't let him become anxious about his talent.

Glandular fever

Although it usually affects children in their teens, this viral infection can also occur in young children. It is passed from person to person through intimate contact allowing exchange of saliva, which is why it is also known as the 'kissing disease'.

Glandular fever has nothing to do with glands but is caused by a virus. It begins in the same way as flu, with a sore throat, aches, pains and tiredness, and may be accompanied by a light rash. Although it is not dangerous, glandular fever is quite debilitating, and may last for some time, with lingering effects still being felt up to six months later. Always consult your doctor for a correct assessment, because the symptoms – fatigue, headaches, fever, sore throat and swollen lymph nodes in the neck, armpits and groin– can mirror those of other complaints. The diagnosis of glandular fever will be confirmed with a blood test.

If your child has a fever, keep him warm and give him lots of liquid to drink. You will need to keep him off school for at least a month, and inform other parents. The virus may reappear in the two years after the first attack, so be watchful for symptoms, and consult your doctor if you are worried.

See also **Fever**

Glue ear

This is a common problem that occurs when sticky fluid builds up in the middle ear cavity, usually in response to a cold or mucus build-up. The Eustachian tube which runs from the ear to the throat becomes blocked and the fluid is unable to drain away. Both ears tend to be affected at the same time, and the symptoms can include earache and impaired hearing. Sometimes the first symptom is slowness of speech.

Doctors will normally prescribe antibiotics in the first instance to see if they clear up the mucus. If this is unsuccessful or if the problem keeps recurring, the surgical insertion of a small grommet to improve drainage may be recommended. Osteopathy – particularly cranio-sacral therapy – can also be very effective in treating glue ear.

> **Caution:** Always have your baby or child's hearing tested after an episode of glue ear.

See also **Earache, Hearing**

Growth

All children grow and put on weight at their own rate. In the first few months of your baby's life, weight gain needs to be carefully monitored to ensure that all is well, but after this it is the regularity of weight gain that is important. Growth charts show the expected ranges of small, medium and large babies, but there is considerable room for personal difference. It is good to use these as a guide, but not to become over-anxious about them. You will get guidance on this from your clinic.

The average newborn baby weighs 3.4 kg (7½ lb), and 95 per cent of babies weigh between 2.5 and 4.3 kg (5–9 lb). Babies often lose up to 10 per cent of their birth weight in the first few days, and this is perfectly natural, and will usually be regained by the end of the second week. Sometimes feeding is difficult at first, or there can be an allergy to formula, and sometimes babies' growth happens in spurts and can be quite irregular. Growth is rapid in the first six months, then it slows down towards the end of the first year. In general a baby of average weight will increase its length by a quarter during the first six months, and double its weight.

Do not worry if your baby gains weight more slowly than you expect him to; you can rely on the clinical checks to ensure that you are getting the support that you need, and can raise any concerns you have with your doctor. Only in extreme circumstances, if your baby continues to fail to thrive, hospitalization may be necessary so that he can be given nutrients and fluids intravenously.

Boys and girls will show different growth spurts, and often grow and develop at different rates throughout their childhood. Always take an individual approach and, assuming that broad health guidelines have been met, try not to make comparisons with others.

Hand–eye co-ordination

Babies start life by using their hands and eyes separately and the art of putting the two together is known as hand–eye co-ordination – an important feature in your child's development that will be used in all sorts of ways. It will help your child translate thoughts into actions, and to implement his desires in a practical way.

Your baby's most obvious first attempts at hand–eye co-ordination will be seen when he reaches out to touch a toy, your face or an object in front of him. Gradually, over time, he will learn to control his hands by watching what he is doing, until it becomes an unconscious act. Baby gyms are a fun way to introduce games that will stimulate hand–eye co-ordination and provide lots of enjoyment at the same time.

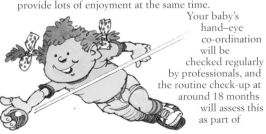

Your baby's hand–eye co-ordination will be checked regularly by professionals, and the routine check-up at around 18 months will assess this as part of observing your child at play. He may, for example, be asked to stack some bricks on a tractor, or build them into a tower.

Crawling improves left and right brain co-ordination and activity, so encourage this as an exercise even after your child is walking on his own. All play activities that improve movement will encourage this facility, and ball games are among the most fun ways to use this skill. Catching a ball that is coming towards him, and learning how to aim it when throwing it back will exercise your child's body well and improve general co-ordination.

See also **Check-ups, Left- or right-handedness, Playing**

Handicaps

Your child will be assessed shortly after birth for any handicap or abnormality, and advice and support will be available through the hospital services.

It is very important for parents of handicapped children to have some help or someone to talk to about their feelings. Support groups and trained counsellors can be invaluable in this respect.

Often potential handicaps can be detected before birth, and full screening services will pick out specific illnesses early in the pregnancy, allowing counselling to come into play at an earlier stage. Certain mental handicaps, on the other hand, may not actually be detected or diagnosed until the child starts school.

A handicap presents a specific challenge to the affected child as well as to his family and carers. Prejudices and ignorance are among the biggest hurdles to be overcome in managing life successfully with disability. Other children should be taught not to laugh at those who are different from themselves.

Hay fever

This seasonal allergic reaction involves a cold-like response to pollen in the air throughout the summer months. Symptoms include:

- runny nose
- sore throat
- sore and red (sometimes swollen) eyes
- a general weariness from the constant sneezing
- feelings of soreness and irritation.

Sneezes and soreness can appear within seconds of exposure to the pollen or grain, and symptoms are often worse in the evenings. A heavy rainfall will temporarily reduce the pollen count.

Symptoms may be alleviated by:

- keeping windows and doors closed, especially in the evening

- screening any open windows with a damp, fine-weave net curtain
- applying a smear of Vaseline to each nostril
- regularly washing hair
- wearing sunglasses
- changing bedding and outdoor clothing regularly
- keeping away from trees and long grasses.

Do not be tempted to dose with over-the-counter anti-histamine medications, but consult your doctor and ask for an individual prescription if symptoms become unmanageable.

See also **Allergies**

Head injuries

Children often bang their heads and are fine and running around again within minutes. If your child complains of a headache after a head injury, move a finger back and forth in front of him and check whether his eyes follow the finger normally. If this is all right, let him rest, well attended, for an hour or so, and if he has not improved after that time, take him to your doctor.

  If there is an open wound, cover any bleeding with a clean pad or handkerchief held tight against it. Check for blood or clear liquid coming from the ears or nose, and place a pad against the ear or nose to absorb it then take your child to the nearest casualty department. Bleeding can seem profuse even from a small wound on the head, and lumps can seem to be very large, so try not to panic.

He should also be taken to casualty if there is:

- dizziness
- vomiting
- loss of consciousness
- light sensitivity
- confusion.

After a bump on the head, watch your child carefully for any change in his behaviour, energy levels or appetite that day and, if in any doubt, take him to be checked by a doctor.

See also **First aid**

Hearing

Newborn babies will be startled by noise, but not usually able to source it until some time later – sometimes as early as one week, but more commonly at around one month. They will then start to recognize familiar sounds, like the sound of their mother's or primary carer's voice, and by about four months will be able to locate a sound and turn towards it. By six months they may be able to differentiate voices and tunes, combine sounds, and know their own name. Hearing development is essential to language skills, so if you suspect any problem, it is important to have it confirmed as early as possible. Look out for:

- inattentiveness
- child becoming easily distracted
- restlessness
- slowness in making sounds
- lack of responsiveness to you
- lack of interest in surroundings.

Older children may mask any deafness quite successfully, but it will show in a slower rate of academic learning. Try testing your baby or young child by approaching him out of his line of sight and calling his name, or simply calling to him. Sit behind him and make a clapping or other moderately loud sound. Hold him and watch television together, then talk to him and see whether he notices both sources of sound. Temporary deafness can occur because of problems with the tonsils or adenoids, from glue ear or cold and mucus congestion.

Your baby will have his hearing tested routinely at around seven months, but if you notice any potential problem at all, you should always contact your doctor straight away.

See also **Glue ear**

Hiccups

Hiccuping is an interruption in the smooth pattern of air flowing in and out of the lungs, caused by regular contractions of the muscular diaphragm. In a new baby it can be a sign that his breathing muscles are getting stronger and trying to work in unison. Babies will often get hiccups after a feed, especially if they were at all rushed, or if not adequately winded afterwards. Young children might suffer similarly after meals. Giving your child a mild fright will often startle him out of an attack, and placing a cold teaspoon on his cheek is one of the best and quickest remedies.

To avoid hiccups, always feed your baby with his upper body slightly raised, and keep him still and upright for a few minutes after each feed. With older children, keep them from running around for at least five minutes after eating, and insist that meals are taken sitting down. A teaspoonful of dry granulated sugar nearly always stops hiccups for older children. If your baby is hiccuping, sit him up and gently rub his back, as though you were winding him. Small sips of gripe water or home-made dill seed tea will help relieve any spasm, but if this is a recurrent problem, you may wish to consider consulting a paediatric osteopath or cranio-sacral therapist for an assessment and treatment of any imbalance of pressures around the diaphragm. This can sometimes become stressed through the birth, and can easily be released with two or three treatment sessions.

Holidays

Babies are relatively portable, while toddlers and young children can be more problematic, but don't let that put you off taking holidays. They just take a little more planning when children are involved.

Self-catering and camping are good options for young families, as they allow children the freedom and informality they need, and may make it easier to maintain household routines like meal-, bath- and bed-times. Most hotels, guest houses and bed and breakfasts will cater for families, however, and it can be a welcome break to have someone else look after the domestic arrangements. Check with the establishment first to ensure it is 'child-friendly'.

Tour operators and airlines usually offer reduced fares for children, but it is important to check this because age limits can vary widely. If you are planning to hire a car, ask for appropriate car seats/boosters to be included (*see also* **Car safety**) and ensure that there will be seat belts in the back.

Wherever you choose to take your holiday, your child will probably need to be given some safety guidelines. Make sure he knows that he should never:

- wander out of sight of you
- go into the sea on his own
- cross a main road by himself
- go into a field with any animals in it
- touch any machinery or equipment.

Much of this is common sense, but it is a good idea to go over it with your child.

If travelling abroad, you should take supplies of any special feed or baby care products with you. It is also useful to know a few key medical phrases in the language of the country you intend to visit, especially if you have any specific concerns, for example if your child is allergic to antibiotics. Essentials also include

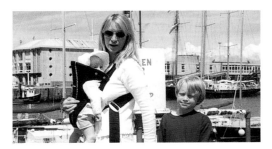

any toys that your child will not sleep without, and his favourite bedtime game or storybooks to help him feel comfortable when he is away.

Consult your doctor if you are planning to travel abroad to areas where inoculations are necessary. It is not usually recommended that babies who are still being breast-fed receive travel inoculations, but individual advice should always be sought.

See also **Car journeys, Drowning, Sunburn, Travel sickness**

Hospital stays

If your child needs to stay in hospital, it may be possible for you to stay with him. Many units keep a dedicated area for parents to stay in; if not you may simply have to sleep in a chair by your child's bed.

Speak to your doctor or one of the nursing sisters before your child is admitted for advice on what to bring with you. It may be that he will need to be kept still and quiet, in which case you could read to him from his favourite story books, or bring some calming but familiar music to listen to. If he is in for observation, or is allowed to be more active, then choose one or two favourite toys.

If you know ahead of time that your child requires a stay in hospital, talk to him about it, and give him as much information as he asks for about what is likely to happen. Tell him in a way that he is able to understand, and answer any questions he may have – your doctor or nurse will be able to help.

If you can't stay with your child in the hospital, double check that the ward sister has your telephone number, and tell your child when you will be back to visit. Although older children may view a short stay in hospital as a bit of an adventure, most will still have some anxieties.

Always take with you:

- your child's nightclothes, dressing gown and slippers
- any favourite sleeping toy or comforter
- his washing items and a towel
- any medication your child is taking (this should be shown to the admitting doctor and the nurse)
- a drawing pad and some coloured pencils.

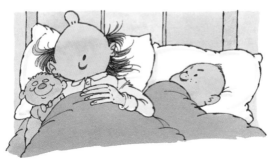

Older children may like to have a disposable camera or a journal, and a small personal radio-cassette player might be useful for playing music or story tapes.

Hygiene

Good hygiene is essential when taking care of your baby or child, and a new arrival to the family provides a good opportunity to review hygiene procedures throughout the house.

Always observe the following basic rules in the kitchen:

- Wash your hands before preparing any food.
- Keep all surfaces clean.
- Change your dishcloths and sponges regularly.
- If you are bottle-feeding you will need to sterilize all equipment.
- Use separate chopping boards for uncooked meat and other foods.
- Never store uncooked meats at the top of the fridge where they could drip onto fresh foods.

Always wash your hands before and after changing your baby, and introduce this habit to them once they are using the toilet themselves, and as a before-meals habit. Review personal hygiene activities such as good dental care and toilet habits so that it will be easy to introduce them to your growing child. Consider medicated hand-washes rather than soap, and use anti-bacterial sprays when cleaning.

Hyperactivity

Some experts believe that hyperactivity is the result of a brain disorder, while others feel it may stem from problems in relating to parents or other carers. There is also research to show that certain foods, drinks and additives can increase hyperactive tendencies in children, and the most common are orange dyes, fizzy drinks and refined sugar.

Symptoms of hyperactivity may include:

- sleeplessness
- disruptive behaviour

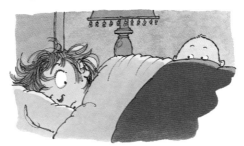

- tantrums
- excitability
- poor attention span
- clumsiness
- learning difficulties
- aggression.

It is worth removing all E numbered additives from your child's diet if there are any signs of energy imbalances. If these are a contributing factor, results can be seen within two to three weeks – sometimes within three days. There is also likely to be an immediate reversion if the food or drink is reintroduced. In some cases drug treatment and/or psychological therapy may be needed.

Check with your doctor that your child's behaviour is not masking a problem such as dyslexia, and develop strategies to cope with challenging behaviours. It is important to remember, however, that a hyperactive child is not being deliberately difficult. Children will often grow out of the symptoms once there are proper channels for their energy so make sure you provide adequate stimulation for a clever child, and plenty of games and activities for a bored one.

Immunization

See **Vaccinations**

Independence

By encouraging your child's efforts and reinforcing his sense of self-worth, you will also be helping him to grow independent.

Babies don't have any real independence from their parents. By the time a child is two years old, he will be showing some signs of independence, and at around four he will be actively testing his ability to be out there on his own, and he will also be flexing some muscle in relationships.

Encourage your child to join in the decision-making process for all matters that concern him directly, like

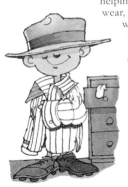

helping to choose what clothes to wear, which shop to go to first, which bedtime story to read together. Help your child to understand his own and other people's feelings so that he is equipped to relate to others, and understand how similar we all are. These measures are as important to your child's growing independence as are more practical things such as teaching him how to tie shoelaces, and speak up in class.

Insomnia

For children. A regular established routine, such as bath, then story, then bed, helps most babies and young children feel comfortable with the bedtime process, so that they get off to sleep easily. A light feed or a milky drink shortly before bed can also be helpful. Gentle rocking, soothing music, the comfort of a familiar toy or story, and time alone with a parent, all set the scene for a restful atmosphere and help prepare your child for sleep.

Encourage your child to start preparing for bed earlier in the evening by slowly quietening down and encouraging more restful activities and pursuits towards bedtime. Try to ensure that he uses up his physical energy during the day, and has plenty of stimulation from activities that will stretch him, so that he is ready for sleep when you want him to be.

If your child suddenly starts being unable to sleep, or if having tried the above strategies your child's not sleeping continues to be an ongoing problem, do check with your GP as there may be more deep-rooted causes. (*See also* **Sleeping problems**)

For adults. Parents often experience insomnia as a reaction to being woken in the night by a baby, and then through caring for young children. Try to re-establish a regular routine, and use your alarm clock to alter your wake-up time by fifteen minutes each morning. Waking up earlier encourages your body clock to re-set itself and in about a month you should find that you are getting to sleep at a reasonable hour.

Left-or right-handedness

Your child may show a preference for using one hand in favour of the other at about eighteen months old.

Left-handedness causes no great difficulty in life – indeed, many great artists, musicians and tennis players are left-handed – and should not be discouraged as was thought in the past. Gadgets such as left-handed scissors can help children with those few tasks that may present a problem, but it will make his life a lot easier if he is also taught to master using scissors with his right-hand from the start

Exercise your child's dexterity, whichever hand he favours, and also give him plenty of opportunity to express his abilities with the hand he uses less. Tell your school if your child favours his left hand, and ensure that they will continue to encourage this.

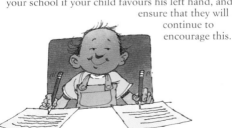

Lying

Children lie for any number of specific reasons, but almost always out of some type of distress or when they are trying to shift blame on to someone else. If you discover your child in a lie, be sensitive but firm. There is no call to shame them, but it is important to address the issue. If your child constructs lies around specific events or situations, this may help you to discover the real cause of the problem.

Some children lie because they are bored and understimulated and need to channel their creativity; others lie to seek attention, as a cry for help, or simply because they wish things were different. Help your child to realize why it is important to know fact from fiction and try to explain the value of trust, and being trustworthy. You will also need to explain that there are different ways of telling the truth, for example how to be truthful without being blunt and hurtful towards other people.

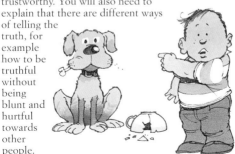

Manual skills

Each time your baby reaches for an object, or moves something from one place to another, he increases his manual ability. By the time he is around nine or ten months he will have developed a 'pincer grip' using his thumb and forefinger, which enables him to pick up small objects.

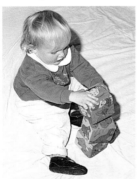

Stimulate his natural inquisitiveness by giving him a wide variety of shapes and textures to explore. Give him shape-sorting toys, and encourage him to hold his own bottle to drink from once he is old enough (around a year), and to feed himself with finger foods. Bricks and stacking beakers are fun to play with and help to develop dexterity, and anything with a screwing action improves his wrist movement. Around 18 months is an ideal time to introduce your child to some chunky crayons and paper, and kneading modelling clay or playdough will also help to develop strength and manipulative skills.

By around three years old your child's manual skills will be sufficiently developed to allow him to zip and unzip his clothing, throw a ball, and draw recognizable shapes.

See also **Check-ups, Hand–eye co-ordination**

Manners

Every family has its own views on how children should and should not behave, and just what social graces are expected of them. As a general rule, 'manners' are based on good sociable behaviours, and if they are practised in the home, it will be natural for children to practise them in the world outside.

The following are generally accepted to be 'good manners' and are worth encouraging in your child:

- saying 'please' and 'thank you'
- covering his mouth when he coughs, and sneezing into a tissue or handkerchief
- deferring to older family members and those in authority

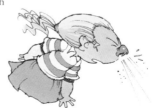

- being polite and considerate to others
- observing good table manners (*see also* **Mealtimes**).

Explain to your child why you feel these things are important, and how they are viewed by outsiders. Let him know, too, that the definition of good manners may differ in other households or cultures.

Massage

Massage is a wonderful way for either parent to 'bond' with a baby. It has also been found to help with problems such as insomnia, headaches, breathing difficulties and poor circulation.

You can massage your baby any time and as often as you like. You do not need to use any special oils or creams; just covering your baby's skin with the lightest touch of your hands will delight him, wake up his nerve endings, and stimulate good feelings. Before you start, make sure that both of you are warm and relaxed.

You will need:

- a pillow, cushion or changing mat to put the baby on (if the weather is cold, place this on a hot water bottle, or wrap one in a towel and put it next to the baby)
- a soft towel or blanket to wrap around the baby

- optional cream or warmed (not hot) oil (this can be a specialist product, or you can use almond, sesame or olive oil from the kitchen; do not use any oil or cream on babies under one month old).

It is best to work on the floor or on a bed or other large area where there is no risk of the baby falling. Start by undressing your baby and letting him enjoy the feeling of the air around him and the freedom to kick and move around. Hold your baby quite close to you so he can see your face, and will be able to communicate with you and maintain eye contact. This is especially important for the first few occasions.

Begin with your baby lying on his back, and simply stroke him. If you are using oil or cream, rub that well into your hands first; never drop it directly onto the baby. Use gentle, continuous strokes to follow the lines of your baby's body. Make sweeping strokes that

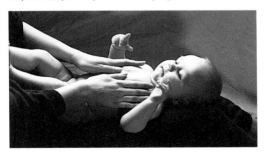

follow on from one another along all the long surfaces
like his arms, then smaller, circular movements around
the joints (like elbows and knees). You can cover the
whole body, starting at the head and working down to
the feet, turning him over or on to his side to work
down his back and head. Make sure that your baby
does not become cold, especially if you have used an
oil or cream to massage him with.

Babies usually love being massaged, and will let you
know quite clearly with their giggles and squeals when
it feels great, and which bits to linger over. Sometimes
the experience will be very relaxing and he may
become quiet or even doze off.

Massage your baby as often as you both enjoy. It
can even become a regular feature in a bath-time or
nappy-changing routine, or a special weekly treat for
you both.

Caution: Do not use adult massage oil blends or
essential oils on your baby without specialist
advice. Do not massage a baby who has a fever,
and avoid any areas that are cut or bruised or
where there is scar tissue.

Mealtimes

Encourage eating together at breakfast and for
weekend meals from as early on as possible. Your child
may be able to enjoy eating with you regularly by the
time he is about four years old. Younger children will

need to eat earlier, and babies and toddlers will require help with managing their meals. A high chair or booster seat and a bib will help to keep mess and fuss to a minimum, as well as making the child more comfortable when eating.

If you have more than one child, keeping order at the table will be as important as the food itself. Teach good table manners as early as possible, and certainly from the age of two, but you'll have to keep reminding them for many years to come. Good manners may include:

• always asking for food to be passed rather than reaching for it;

• staying seated at the table and not leaving until the meal is over;

• learning the correct cutlery to use for each course, and how to use it;

• refraining from food-throwing.

Regular mealtimes are an important part of ensuring your child's health. His body needs fuel at

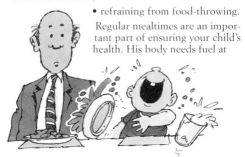

regular intervals that he can depend on, and this also introduces a valuable element of routine into his life. Studies show that children who eat breakfast perform better physically and mentally than those who do not. If your child is eating nutritious meals there will be less likelihood of him eating unhealthy snacks.

Give your child his evening meal at least two hours before bedtime, but if he has trouble getting off to sleep, or feels hungry before bed, a milky drink and a light snack will usually fill the gap.

See also **Eating problems, Nutrition**

Measles

This is a highly contagious, childhood illness, but one that is far less common than it once was due to immunization (although most children who do catch measles have, in fact, been vaccinated).

Symptoms of measles seem like those of a cold or flu, until a brownish red rash starts to cover the upper body. A raised temperature, and chest or ear infections may develop, alongside enlarged lymph nodes and feelings of discomfort and irritability. Complications are rare, but include middle ear infection, conjunctivitis, pneumonia and encephalitis.

Give your child plenty to drink and once the diagnosis has been confirmed, keep him away from other children. Keep his temperature down by sponging with tepid water, and occupy him with gentle activities like story-telling and I-spy games. Soak your child in an oatmeal bath to relieve itching, and increase vitamin C in the diet.

> **Caution:** Early diagnosis is important because the rash, raised temperature and flu-like symptoms may indicate other diseases, including meningitis.
>   Get medical help immediately if your child's breathing becomes shallow, if he has any chest pain, or if his temperature rises above 40° C (104° F).

See also **Vaccinations**

Meningitis

Meningitis is an inflammation of the coverings of the brain. If it is picked up early enough it can be treated successfully, but the onset can be very rapid and it is a very dangerous condition. There are several types of meningitis, some of which can be vaccinated against.

In babies under 12 months, look for the following symptoms:

• fever

• a high-pitched, moaning cry

• difficulty in waking

• refusal to feed

• pale and blotchy skin

- red or purple spots that do not fade under pressure. (Press the side of a glass against the rash to see if it fades and loses colour. Contact your doctor immediately if it does not.)

In older children look for the following:

- red or purple spots (do the 'glass test' as above)

- stiffness in the neck

- drowsiness/confusion

- severe headache

- sore throat

- photophobia (dislike of bright light).

Contact your doctor urgently if your child is ill with one or more of the above. If you are still worried after seeking advice, trust your instincts and take your child to the nearest casualty department.

See also **Vaccinations**

Moodiness

Most moodiness is harmless, but it can be a sign of ill health, and may be the first signal of any number of complaints from a cold to the measles. If it is uncharacteristic, and there is no obvious sign of illness, check your child's diet, and consider reducing refined sugar, artificial colourings (especially orange), and all E numbers. Depending on the age of your child, check whether he might have had access to any mood-altering substances, either at home or at school. It is also worth checking that an upset to his routine hasn't unsettled him, or that this might not be anything more sinister than a normal reaction to changes in his emotional world, such as family members leaving, or joining the household.

Consult your doctor if symptoms do not resolve.

Mouth-to-mouth resuscitation

See **First aid**

Mumps

This is a viral illness affecting children mainly between the ages of four and fourteen, although it can be prevented by immunization. It causes swelling in the salivary glands on each side of the jaw making it difficult to swallow, and even to talk. There may also be flu-like symptoms including a headache, and a raised temperature. Your child is likely to feel unwell for a few days before the symptoms appear and there will be accompanying soreness in the testicles for older boys and in the abdomen for girls.

Offer your child lots of easy-to-swallow drinks, juices and liquidized soups. Ice cream and milkshakes will help to ease the discomfort. Make sure you monitor his temperature and bathe him with tepid water if it becomes raised. Place a covered hot water bottle against the worst affected side of the face, and make sure he has plenty of bed rest.

> **Caution:** Always have your doctor confirm this diagnosis and consult him again if symptoms persist for more than ten days, and if there is any worsening of headache, or neck stiffness. This could be the sign of serious complications such as meningitis or encephalitis. If contracted in adulthood mumps can also cause inflammation of the ovaries in women and the testicles in men which can result in fertility problems.

See also **Vaccinations**

Nappies

Your child will be in nappies until he is fully potty-trained. There is a range of nappy options, and although most parents use disposables, you can also choose terry cotton and shaped reusables.

TERRY COTTON

Advantages
Made from natural fibre,
and may be kinder to
the skin;
environmentally
friendly.

Disadvantages
You will use more
detergent and energy to
wash them; they will
need to be soaked and
boil washed.

SHAPED REUSABLES

Advantages
Less bulky than a terry;
environmentally
friendly.

Disadvantages
Expensive; less power of
absorption than terry-
towelling nappies

DISPOSABLES

Advantages
Easy to use; readily
available; come in a
range of fittings to
ensure maximum
comfort.

Disadvantages
Not bio-degradable;
expensive.

CHANGING NAPPIES

Bulky nappies can restrict movement and they may
impede your child in learning to walk. There are now
smaller disposable nappies available for play and
activity times.

You will need to change your baby's nappy regularly: expect to change a newborn's nappy after each feed.

To change your baby you will need:

- changing mat or comfortable, wipe-clean surface
- towel or cloth
- baby wipes or cotton wool and cleanser or water for cleaning
- oil, lotion or powder (*see also* **Nappy rash**)
- fresh nappy
- container for the soiled nappy.

Lay your baby down on his back, and make eye contact with him. Remove a layer of clothing, and loosen the old nappy. Hold your baby by the ankles, and gently lift his bottom up off the surface. This will enable you to remove the soiled nappy with your other hand. Allow him some freedom to roll around (always watching if he is on a raised surface) or kick his legs while you reach for a baby wipe (or cotton wool and water) to clean him. Spread out the fresh nappy; lift your baby again by the ankles, and position it under him; secure the nappy in place before putting his clothes back on.

Nappy rash

This sore, red rash can be very irritating for your baby, and can sting and burn him each time he urinates or fills his nappy. It can develop very quickly, and needs prompt attention.

Protect against nappy rash by applying a barrier cream to the skin around your baby's bottom and thighs at each nappy change. This is much more effective and safer than talcum powder which can

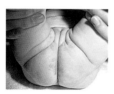

chafe and cause breathing difficulties if inhaled.

Let the air get to your baby's bottom by leaving his nappy off as much as possible, and guard against dampness by frequent changing.

Nosebleeds

These can be a common response to a knock on the nose, continuous picking and prodding, hard blowing or catarrh. They often stop quite quickly, although the amount and flow of blood can seem alarming. Address any boisterousness or co-ordination problems if your child seems to be knocking himself a lot.

When a bleed occurs, lean your child over the sink or bowl and pinch his nostrils together, or press a bunched-up tissue firmly against the affected side, for ten minutes. Encourage him to spit out any blood rather than swallowing it. A cold compress (a clean tea-towel wrung under the cold tap) placed on the back of the neck will cool and soothe the child, and may lessen the bleeding. Stay with your child and comfort him, and do not allow him to blow his nose again until all bleeding is stopped and any dry blood around the nostrils has fallen off.

> **Caution:** Consult your doctor if the bleeding lasts for more than fifteen minutes, or if nosebleeds occur frequently.

Nutrition

The food you give your child is the building material for his growing body, and its quality needs to be the best you can provide.

Your child needs a good balance of protein, carbohydrates, vitamins, minerals, and trace elements. You will also need to make decisions about whether and when to introduce animal protein, and other complex foods such as wheat and dairy products. Your health visitor will be experienced with infant nutrition and can help you to come up with an eating plan that will relieve you of worry and provide your child with all his needs. Ensure that your child's diet is as varied as possible.

Do not routinely give your child vitamin drops or other dietary supplements unless advised to do so by a health professional.

Nutritional guidelines to follow when shopping:

• Consider choosing organically grown foods.

• Always read the labels of any prepared foods so that you can eliminate harmful E numbers and additives.

• Limit the amount of refined sugar you give your child, and keep added salt to a minimum.

See also **E numbers, First foods, Mealtimes**

Only children

Only children have special needs. Because there are no siblings to deflect the focus of parents, and to learn about relationships with, they tend to be more independent, yet at the same time they can be insecure. It is important to provide social experiences for only children from well before school age.

Developing the imagination is rarely a difficulty with only children, although it is most important that they learn to communicate effectively in as many media as possible, and they should be encouraged to translate their fantasies into physical reality, for example painting, drawing, writing and making music.

Encourage your only child to establish friendships from among his own peer group, and make sure he has plenty of stimulation and activities at home to prevent boredom from setting in.

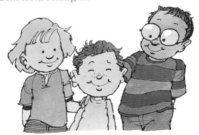

Pets

These make wonderful companions for slightly older children, and can be an excellent way to introduce them to the concepts of responsibility and care, as well as providing a good leisure time activity.

• Take care in your choice of pets, and make sure that they are appropriate for your child's age.

- Dogs should be trained before the arrival of a baby.
- Cats should never be left alone with babies – there is a possibility that they will sit on and suffocate them.
- Birds can present a health hazard; they must be kept in cages and out of reach of growing children.

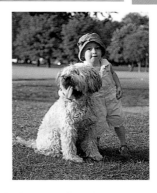

- Fish tanks must also be kept out of reach and securely covered.
- Cages must be kept safe from prying fingers.
- All pets must be checked regularly by a vet and should be dewormed or deloused as necessary.
- Children must be taught to wash their hands after touching their pets.

When your child is old enough you can teach him how to groom, feed and water his pets.

Always teach your child to be extra careful around other people's pets as some animals can react with aggression to strangers.

See also **Worms**

Playing

Every area of your child's learning can be reinforced through some form of play, whether it is movement through dancing along with you, or hand–eye co-ordination through playing with a ball.

Here are some ideas and guidelines for play:

- *Drawing and painting* can provide endless entertainment from around 18 months. Always choose non-toxic paints, pencils and crayons.
- *Pretend-cooking and dressing up games* develop your child's imagination from around 18 months.
- *Books*: even small babies enjoy looking at picture books. Your local library will have a good selection of children's books and may run story sessions.
- *Playing with water* (always supervised) is fun for all ages.

See also **Hand–eye co-ordination, Manual skills, Toys**

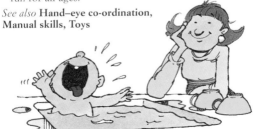

Post-natal depression

Probably two-thirds of mothers get the 'blues' around four to five days after childbirth, caused mainly by exhaustion and hormonal changes. For some women this depression becomes severe and persistent and it is important that they seek help from a GP or health visitor. Left untreated, post-natal depression can prevent you from bonding well with your new baby and put pressure on other relationships in the family.

Potty training

This is an important milestone in your child's development, so take the time to ensure it is as relaxed and untraumatic as possible.

By about two years old, your toddler's muscles will have developed enough for him to know when he wants to use the toilet – until then he may have had some awareness without being able to control it. By three years old most children will be dry through the day, and many will be dry through the night too, but you will need to be prepared for the odd accident, especially during exciting or stressful times.

Try the following strategies:
• Let your child play with a thoroughly cleaned potty when very young. Once he gets to know it, and is

comfortable with it, you can begin to explain what it is for. Be prepared to repeat this several times.

- Get him used to sitting on the potty. Do this several times a day, and always praise him for sitting on it.
- Read to your child while he is on the potty, let him flick through books himself or sing songs together – anything to make potty-time fun.
- Praise your child generously for any success with the potty.
- After a few successes let your child run around without a nappy for short periods each day. This will make it easier for him to get to his potty on time, but you must be prepared for a few accidents.

Do not try to potty train when your child is too young or clearly unready, and don't give up too quickly; it is a project that requires some patience. Children will have different needs, too; some prefer potty time to be private, while others will be proud of their efforts, and be happy to sit in the middle of the room. Do not hurry your child.

Some children bypass the potty altogether and feel

more comfortable with a toilet. You can buy special children's toilet seats and a plastic 'step' for standing on to reach the right height.

Your own attitude to the toilet will influence your child's development. If he is free to come into the bathroom with you, and you are easy and relaxed about physical functions, he is more likely to be the same. Boys especially will want to stand 'like Daddy', and if going into the toilet with him is a possibility, it will help to build a young boy's confidence.

Don't try to train your child at night time until he is clean and dry during the day and has been for some time. Waking up with dry nappies can be an indication that he is ready for the next step but, once again, you must be prepared for accidents.

Rashes

These can appear for any number of reasons, often as an allergic response to some type of food or contact, or as an early sign of an illness such as measles, especially when accompanied by a raised temperature.

If your baby or child develops a rash whose cause is unknown, consult your doctor straight away. Otherwise, if you know the cause, for example your child may have just fallen into some nettles, treat the skin with an oatmeal bath or camomile lotion to soothe it. Keep hands clean and nails short to discourage breaking the skin if scratched.

Caution: If your child is vomiting, and has a high fever or headache, consult your doctor straight away. Some foods, such as shellfish, can cause life-threatening reactions. If your child develops a rash immediately after eating something, take him to the casualty department straight away.

See also **Allergies, Fever, Measles, Meningitis, Rubella**

Reading and writing

Encourage your child to follow his own curiosity about reading and writing. There is much satisfaction to be had from forming letters, and spelling out words, and these can become part of your child's range of abilities even before he goes to school. Reading to him from a very early age, and letting him see you reading, will stimulate his interest.

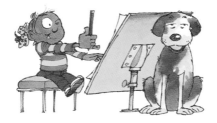

Do not push your child, but respond to any desire to know and do more. Reading heavily illustrated books to him with lots of repeated text will encourage him through word recognition and association with pictures. Younger children particularly enjoy the familiarity of nursery rhyme and song books, and making this part of a bedtime routine will make it an even more comfortable and positive experience.

Once your child can hold a pencil, around the age of 18 months, encourage him to draw pictures and shapes. Once he can make a circle, he is ready to experiment with forming letters which are, after all, just shapes.

Routine

Routine can be as important for adults as it is for babies and children. An established system helps parents feel 'on top of things', and better equipped to deal with the day-to-day complications that parenthood can throw at them.

Newborns do little beyond eating and sleeping but they still respond well to a routine that lets them relax in the subconscious knowledge that you will be providing all their needs. Likewise older babies and children find comfort in a reliable routine.

• Routines should be fun, and logical too – bath-time needs to be close to bedtime, otherwise your child will probably go and get dirty all over again.

- Regular mealtimes will comfort your child, as well as providing his body with the physical energy it needs at good, regular intervals.

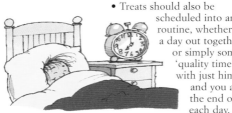

- Treats should also be scheduled into any routine, whether it is a day out together or simply some 'quality time' with just him and you at the end of each day.

See also **Bathing babies and children, Bottle-feeding, Breast-feeding, Mealtimes, Sleep patterns**

Rubella

Also known as German measles, this mild, infectious disease is caused by a virus. Symptoms are a pink rash that usually starts behind the ears and spreads to the forehead, then down over the rest of the body. Your child may also have a slightly raised temperature, and there are usually swollen lymph nodes ('glands') at the back of the neck. He is likely to feel uncomfortable and a little out of sorts, and will need to be kept away from other children and in particular pregnant women as rubella can affect a growing fetus, leading to birth defects such as blindness and deafness. Immunization is now available, however, which gives women who are not already pregnant life-long immunity.

The virus has an incubation period of 14–21 days, and your child can be infectious for up to eight days after the rash appears. Treat your child gently with bed rest and lots of fluids, and keep a watch on his temperature.

> **Caution:** Your doctor will need to confirm the diagnosis and if your child complains of a stiff neck or headache at any time, consult your doctor again immediately.

See also **Vaccinations**

Safety

Your child's security and safety are your responsibility. You should try to instil in him an awareness of safety as early as possible. This might include:

- how to cross a road safely

- coping in other environments, such as when visiting friends and family; this may include a first encounter with domestic pets, or flights of stairs

- asking for help – who to go to if he cannot ask you, how to recognize the people who can help, such as police in uniform and first-aid workers

• what to do if he is separated from you: knowing his address and phone number, or knowing where-abouts he is can be useful in such situations.

It is also important to teach your child how to recognize when something feels uncomfortable or bad, and to practise strategies and ways of saying 'no', and to tell you or whoever is in charge. He needs to know that it is not safe to go for a walk with a stranger, take sweets or gifts from someone he does not know, or get into a car or accept a lift from anyone without your agreement. Alert your child to potential dangers, but try not to frighten him, so that he feels confident and aware, but not intimidated.

Safety in the home with a small baby or child is also vital. You should:

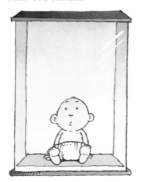

• Fit gates with an automatic lock on any stairs;

• Cover low-level electricity sockets;

• Make sure wires and cables are hidden;

• Fit window locks;

• Move ornaments and houseplants out of reach;

• Fit a fire guard or radiator shields;

- Remove toxic chemicals (bleach, etc.) from within reach and place in a lockable box or cupboard;
- Fit childproof locks on washing machines and other pieces of equipment;
- Avoid accidents in the kitchen – always leave pan handles facing inward and use a stove guard.

If you have a garden you will need to do a safety check there too: get to know poisonous plants and make sure you remove any from your garden; fit a good lock to the entrance gate, and make sure you use it; cover any water feature with strong wire mesh, or fence it off.

See also **Car safety**

Separation anxiety

Always let your child know if you are going to be apart from him for any length of time, and tell him when you expect to be back. Be as specific as possible – 'soon' is too abstract for most children, but they will understand 'by the time you have finished ...' or similarly exact time-periods. Some children will show little interest in your leaving, but may express concern or anxiety once they notice that you are not around; others may be distressed when you leave but are very quickly and easily distracted.

More serious anxiety could lead to your child not wanting to be separated from you at all, and becoming extremely distressed at the prospect of any time apart.

Practise spending time just out of his line of vision, then extend that to being in the next room, and so on. Talk to your child, if he is old enough, to ensure that there are no other reasons for his concerns, and check that he is not unhappy with the person he is being left with.

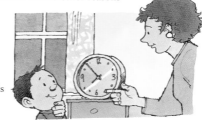

Sex differences

Children tend to develop at different rates. Girls show ability in speaking and communication skills earlier than boys, whereas boys often crawl and walk earlier than girls. Cultural differences figure large, and much depends on how we treat children, and on the models we provide for them. Boys can appear to be more fearless, although girls will often be braver in terms of risk-taking and trying new things, possibly because they feel more confident in their relationship skills.

Many boys seem to enjoy active games and rough and tumble play, while many girls excel at games involving fantasy and imagination, as well as those that are relationship-based or involve caring. These tend to direct us towards choosing ball games for boys and board games for girls, but given the freedom to choose, children will often surprise you with their actual preferences.

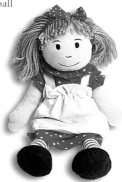

Different areas of a child's personality can be developed by certain toys and activities regardless of their sex and the last thing you should do is worry if your son decides he likes playing with dolls while your daughter prefers trucks.

Shoes

Your child should not wear proper shoes until he can walk alone, and they should only be used for outdoor wear at first.

The bones in a child's foot remain pliable until puberty, and are very easy to pour into misshapen shoes. It is therefore best to have your baby's feet measured by a trained fitter in a children's shoe shop. As a general rule, shoes should be about 1 cm beyond the longest toe in length and wide enough for all the toes to lie flat. Choose shoes with laces, buckles or velcro which will hold the heel in place and stop the foot from slipping forward and damaging the toes.

Have your child's shoe size checked regularly and be prepared for him to grow out of his shoes very quickly – as often as every three months. It is also important for socks to be the right size.

> Consult your GP if you have any concerns about your child's feet and he or she will refer you to a chiropodist, orthopaedic surgeon, paediatrician, or paediatric physiotherapist if necessary.

Shyness

Some children will never be as outgoing as others, and there is a lot to be said for not being brash or too demanding. If your child is shy, give him time to come out of his shell, and find as many ways as you can to boost his confidence through praise, and through creating lots of experiences and situations in which he can do well. Try not to be too protective because sometimes dealing with situations on his own will reinforce your child's confidence.

Introducing a shy child to a playgroup or nursery will be easier if you talk to him about it first and take time to prepare him for what he is likely to experience, presenting it in as positive a light as possible. It is a good idea to let nursery or other teachers know if your child is timid or shy, as they will have experience in encouraging and helping children like this. Most children will take about a month to settle in to a new situation or environment, but your child may take a little longer if he is not used to being around other children. Do not worry unduly. It seems that shyness is a genetic predisposition, so you or your partner may well find some good coping mechanisms if you delve into your memory.

Sibling rivalry

Children often feel threatened when faced with someone who is going to be competing for their parents' love and care. Preparing your child for a new arrival will go a long way towards reassuring him. Children over two will to some extent be able to become involved with and learn from the pregnancy, and this will make them feel more connected with their younger brother or sister when they arrive.

Once the new baby arrives, make special time for your existing child or children, and try to include them in family activities so that the focus is not entirely on the new child. Similarly, if merging families, or entering an extended family situation, try to allow as much preparation time as possible, and continue to reinforce your individual, special relationship with each child.

It can be difficult for parents to treat (or be seen to treat) each child as fairly as possible and this can become a breeding ground for jealousy or resentment. Try to explain, particularly to slightly older children, that treating them 'fairly' does not always mean treating them the same, and that age differences must be reflected in both treats and responsibilities.

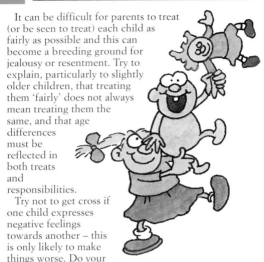

Try not to get cross if one child expresses negative feelings towards another – this is only likely to make things worse. Do your best to defuse the situation, and make some individual time for both children.

You might also reinforce the fact that everyone has different skills and attributes, likes different things and responds in different ways, and that each person's relationship with another person will be different in some ways.

Encourage your children to express and discuss their feelings – the earlier these things are dealt with in the

family, the lower the risk of family feuds and
individual insecurities.

See also **Fighting, Smacking**

Sleep patterns

In the first few months, your baby is likely to sleep for
about four hours at a time during the night before
waking, usually with hunger. Over the next month,
that usually extends to five hours, and it can be up to a
year (although it may be much sooner) before he will
sleep for six hours or through the night. Some children
need an afternoon nap, and others simply will not
settle if put down in the day. The latter are most likely
to sleep right through the night, which is a tremendous
boon.

If your baby sleeps through the night, do not wake
him up to feed him just because in theory he should
eat every so many hours. Likewise, if your toddler
doesn't take an afternoon nap, do not force him to –
he will probably compensate at night.

Children need to be put to bed at a regular time each
evening. Make sure that you have a quiet wind-down
before trying to put them to bed. Let your child know
that he can always come to you if he has a problem in
the night, but encourage him to sleep through till
morning. Make mornings fun and active, and encourage
your child to expend his energy in physical ways.

See also **Sleeping problems**

Sleeping problems

Babies: Controlled crying is a specific technique used to address sleeping problems in babies if they often wake in the night crying but you cannot identify any cause. It can be used for babies over six months old and is a way of retraining your baby. Usually things have to get very bad before parents do this, but some babies cry all the time at night and there comes a point when it is inadvisable for parents to go without uninterrupted sleep for any longer.

Before embarking on a controlled crying strategy, have your baby checked over by your GP to ensure that there is no underlying physical cause for his crying. If you decide to go ahead, plan it for a long weekend if you can, when you will not have to cope with the demands of work in the morning.

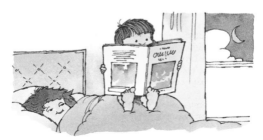

- When your baby cries, make sure that he has had enough to eat and drink, that he is clean and comfortable, and that the room is not too hot or cold.

- Pick him up very briefly, say something comforting so that he hears the sound of your voice, and feels reassured that you came when he cried, then leave the room. He will probably scream at not having the usual cuddles, so try to go just out of earshot, and distract yourself.

- If he is still crying after five minutes, go back to him, say your goodnight words again, but do not pick him up this time or cuddle him.

- Keep this up, every five minutes, until he goes to sleep. If you feel more comfortable, you can stretch the time to ten or even fifteen minutes. If your baby needs changing, do this carefully but without any extra cuddles, and keep the light low, and return him to bed with a minimum of fuss.

It can be very hard not to comfort your baby physically, but you are trying to teach him that he can feel secure without being picked up. For this method to be effective you must see it through. If you give in after an hour, your baby will have learned that to get a cuddle, he just needs to cry for longer.

Children: Some children who are hyperactive or who have attention deficit problems experience sleep disorders as one of their symptoms, and this should be addressed by a consultant or GP. Other children simply have difficulty in sleeping – often because they are unable to switch off and relax, or after a cold or other illness has disrupted their sleep pattern. An excess of sugar, additives, and other stimulants in the diet can make it hard to get to sleep. Carbonated drinks, sweets, puddings, biscuits, desserts and chocolates should all be confined to early in the day, or better still cut out altogether.

Make sure that your child has plenty of opportunity during the day to burn up his physical energy. Explain to your child what sleep is and why he needs it.

If your child has trouble sleeping:

- leave a nearby light on if he is worried about being alone in the dark;

- discourage TV or video viewing for at least an hour before bedtime;

- avoid playing with him if he wakes in the night and don't sit with him until he goes to sleep;

- avoid comforters and putting your child to bed with a bottle, as they encourage bacteria to grow in his mouth and may also cause him to wake more;

- check that the room is dark enough for him (although older children might like a soft light nearby), that he is not too hot or too cold, and that nothing is irritating him, such as a scratchy sheet or hard pillow;

- make sure that the room is adequately ventilated, but that there is no draught;

- ensure that the room is vacuumed regularly, and smoke-free – smoke, and even perfume and dust, can all irritate tiny nasal passages and make breathing difficult.

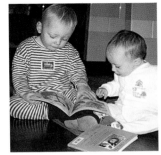

Some children simply do not need very much sleep. If this is the case with your child, and he is not suffering in any way from having less sleep than other children or members of the family, then make sure he has a wide variety of things that he can safely and productively do on his own in bed.

See also **E Numbers, Hyperactivity, Routine**

Slow learners

All children have their own pace, style and limitations. If your child is slow in developing one aspect of his skills, there may be no cause for concern. Individual attention and instruction will often be enough to encourage learning, and redress any imbalance.

It is important that you check for any treatable conditions such as poor eyesight and hearing. Your local education authority will have a special needs department which can help in identifying problems such as dyslexia. They will also be able to provide information and support.

Your child's learning will suffer if he is not happy in a situation, so check too whether he likes his teacher, or if he is being bullied or excluded at school.

If you notice other behavioural difficulties besides an apparent slowness in learning, or if your child seems withdrawn, it is important to discuss this with your doctor. Medical conditions such as autism can manifest in different ways and your doctor will be able to diagnose this properly. **Hyperactivity** (*see* page 114) can also cause learning difficulties, and again, this is something that will need specialist individual attention.

Smacking

Some parents believe that smacking can deter certain repeated behaviours, and that incidents will be retained in the child's memory if they are associated with smacking as a punishment. Some people also hold that it is a fast and effective attention-grabber for a child in a potentially dangerous situation. On the whole, however, it is not a favourable way of asserting authority or commanding respect, and can even show a lack of control. While it may provide temporary relief for the adult, it is passing on the message to the child that violence is acceptable.

If you find your child smacking his friends, he may have learned to do so from watching others or through being smacked himself, or he may simply be experimenting. It is important to teach your child other ways of taking control of his feelings, for getting attention, or expressing frustration and anger.

Equally, if your child is being smacked by another child, he must know that he needs to call for help, or tell whoever is taking care of him right away. Children who are hurting each other in this way should be separated, and talked to individually.

The best tactic when a child is misbehaving is to remove him from the scene immediately so he can't continue. You may decide to put him in a separate room to calm down for a while and then explain to him later exactly what he did wrong.

See also **Discipline, Fighting**

Sore throat

This could be a symptom of a cold or flu, or a more serious complaint such as mumps or tonsillitis.

If your child has a sore throat, make sure he gets plenty of rest and lots to drink. Choose drinks that are non-acidic such as fruit juices diluted half and half with water, or warm milk with a little cinnamon and honey. Liquidize meals if your child is hungry but it hurts too much to eat.

If your child's sore throat is accompanied by any or all of a raised temperature, a rash, swollen lymph nodes, earache, or if the sore throat continues for more than three days, you should contact your doctor.

See also **Colds, Mumps**

Speech

Your baby will probably be making cooing noises and babbling by about three months, but he will have been communicating with you long before then through gestures and movements. By five months he will be using speech-like sounds, and by six months he may respond to his name and combine simple sounds.

By around nine months, one meaningful word may be heard (it may be Mama, or Dada, but these could be used to refer to any number of people or objects; or it may even be 'Spot' if the dog's name is used a lot!). By 11 months he may be using simple words such as 'No' and 'Bye', although again not necessarily in appropriate ways. By the time your child is around 15 months old, he could be expected to use a small vocabulary of up to 20 words that can be completely understood, and be able to put two words together in a sentence. By 18 months your child may well be making himself understood, with a vocabulary of up to 50 words. Boys tend to be slower than girls at picking up language skills.

Young children often substitute a sound they can make for one they can't yet manage, so you may have to learn your toddler's language in order to understand him. The more your child hears the spoken word and has 'conversations' with you and other people, however simple, the more adept his language skills will become. Ensure you develop them as much as you can by talking to your child whenever possible, explaining to him what is going on, naming things, and talking about how they work. All children develop speech at their own rate, but if you have any concerns or anxieties about your child's progress then check with your GP, clinic or health visitor.

Note: Dentists, doctors, and pre-school or nursery teachers should be able to spot any speech abnormalities, but look out for them yourself. If you notice your child lisping or stuttering, seek out a good speech therapist who is used to working with children and will find fun ways to overcome any difficulties. *See also* **Stammering**

Stammering

Stammering, or stuttering, is a common and transitory problem for many two- to three-year-olds who are developing language skills, and want to say much more than they actually can. It also sometimes appears in response to change and emotional upsets, such as the birth of a new baby or parental separation, and can also be a sign of loss of confidence, or even dental problems. Most children grow out of it.

If it persists beyond the age of four, check with your GP who may refer your child to a speech therapist with experience in working with children. Your child's response may be slow, but try not to be impatient. It can be very frustrating for a child who wants to express himself, but finds that he is unable to do so, and it is important that this is addressed so that he does not resort to temper tantrums and other destructive behaviours instead. Sometimes it can be best to leave therapy until the child is at least five.

Do not ask your child to repeat himself more than is absolutely necessary, and try not to say the words for him as this can undermine his confidence still further. Stammers can disappear when he is singing. Imaginary games and acting will allow your child to adopt a different persona, in which the stammer might also disappear.

Sticky eye

Sticky eye is very common in the first few weeks of life, and is often caused by some irritation during delivery. Your baby's eye will ooze and it will be difficult to open after sleeping. It is not serious, but it is important to ensure that the eyes do not become infected.

Clean the affected eye regularly with warm boiled water and a small piece of cotton wool or soft cotton cloth. Always use a separate piece of cotton wool for each eye if both are affected. If you are breast-feeding, increase the amount of vitamin C in your diet, in order to pass it on to your baby and help him to fight any infection. Change bedding and towels frequently. Sticky eye may also be caused by a blocked tear duct. Pressing a finger-tip between the inner corner of the eye and the nose may correct it.

> **Caution:** Contact your doctor or an ophthalmologist if the condition does not clear up.

Stings

If your child is stung by an insect, always try to establish what type of insect it was. Remove the sting if it is sticking out of the skin, by scraping it off. Do not use tweezers. Wash the area with a dilution of vinegar for wasp stings, bicarbonate of soda for bee stings.

Nettle and other plant stings will tend to cover a larger area. Treat by bathing with disinfectant and apply some aloe vera or calamine lotion to soothe the skin. Over-the-counter creams can also be invaluable. If the stinging is severe, treat your child for shock, keeping him warm and cosy and giving him a hot, sweet drink.

> **Caution:** In very rare cases your baby or child may show a strong allergic reaction to a sting, usually the second time he is stung. If your child shows swelling anywhere on his body, or starts to feel light-headed, or has difficulty breathing, take him to hospital straight away to be treated for anaphylactic shock.

Stomach ache

This is a child's most commonly used excuse for not doing something – like going to nursery or school, or carrying out a chore. It is hard to ascertain whether there is a genuine problem, but it can be helpful to check that he has not eaten something and reacted badly to it, or been injured through a fall.

Check his temperature and, if it is raised or if he seems poorly or irritated at all, tuck him up in bed and give him lots of fluids to drink. Check his bowel movements for any irregularity, and monitor him for a day or two. If the pain worsens, contact your GP.

Caution: If the pain persists, or the muscles harden and guard the area when you touch it, or if it is on one side of the abdomen, get your GP to check it straight away. There are causes, such as appendicitis, which will need to be diagnosed straight away and require further treatment.

Suffocation

Suffocation or near-suffocating happens when the nose and mouth are blocked, preventing breathing. This causes asphyxiation (lack of oxygen in the blood).

Teach your child that plastic bags are not playthings, and he is not to put his head (or anyone else's) inside them. Babies and children can suffocate when pillows, bedding, or clothing cover their face, because of a weight on their chest, through breathing in smoke, or being unable to breathe in because of an asthma attack. Quickly remove any obstacle or obstruction, and cradle the child in your arms if he is breathing, while you call for help. If he is not breathing, you need to perform artificial respiration (*see* **First aid**, page 88).

Sunburn

Babies and children can burn very easily, and it is essential that you protect them from the sun. Young skin is particularly at risk from sun damage which can lead to skin cancers. It doesn't mean you need to keep them indoors in hot weather – just follow these rules:

- Always shield babies, even early in the year or in the mornings when the sun is not at its hottest. If you leave your baby in his pram, make sure a parasol or sunshield is fitted, and put a bonnet on his head.

- Children should always wear a hat or stay in the shade.

- Always use sunscreen, and keep your child loosely covered. Choose total sunblock, or the highest factor sunscreen (you can buy ones specially formulated for children) and apply as directed. You may need to reapply this as often as every hour if your child is running around and sweating it off, or playing in a paddling pool; otherwise reapply every three hours.

Treat sunburn straight away by cooling with a compress, dilute vinegar wash, or calamine lotion or

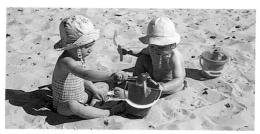

natural yoghurt straight from the fridge. Clothe your child as lightly as possible, or not at all, and use thin cotton sheets on his bed. Keep your child out of the sun for 48 hours after burning.

> **Caution:** Call your doctor if the burning is bad, or covers a large part of the body, and if there is accompanying feverishness and your child seems generally unwell, confused, or drowsy.

Swallowed objects

Unless you actually see your child swallow an object, there may be no sign at all until the object gets into the digestive tract causing a blockage with pain and bloating in the tummy.

   If the object was small and there is no adverse reaction, there is no need to do anything – it will probably pass out the other end. This does not apply to batteries, however, which can be harmful however small, as some can leak. In such a case take your child straight to hospital. Likewise if a sharp object has been swallowed.

   If your child is coughing, encourage him to continue as this may dislodge the object, but if he is **choking** (*see* page 49) and therefore unable to breathe, urgent action is called for. Look in his throat and see if you can easily remove the object with your fingers. If you can't easily remove it do the following:

- Hold a baby firmly along one arm with his head pointing downwards, supporting his jaw with your hand, while you tap him firmly between the shoulder blades to clear the obstruction.

- Hold a small child across your knees with his head and chest hanging over your legs, and again tap him between the shoulder blades. Repeat several times if necessary. If this does not work you will need to try the Heimlich manoeuvre (*see* **First aid,** page 89).

If your child swallows any harmful liquids, do not attempt to treat him, but take him, and the container, to your nearest doctor or hospital.

Safeguards to employ at home include:
- making sure cleaning liquids and fluids are stored well out of reach or in locked cupboards;
- keeping medication clearly labelled and out of reach of all children;
- regularly checking the integrity of door handles, screws, skirting boards and everything else accessible to your child;
- not leaving children unattended in the garden;
- hoovering regularly to keep floor surfaces free from intriguing little objects.

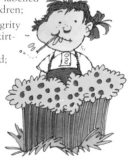

Caution: Children often place small objects in other orifices too, and it is not uncommon to find that beads, small shells, and so forth have been placed in ears and up noses. Blowing the nose into a tissue should dislodge anything stuck up there. Laying the child down on his side may help an object to fall out of his ear; otherwise gently warm a teaspoon of almond or olive oil and, having checked it is not hot, pour it into the outer ear, and the object may just float up and out. Never poke at a stuck object with a cotton bud or anything else. If these methods do not work, take your child to your local hospital, or to your GP straight away.

Swimming

It is a good idea to teach your child to swim as early as possible. It's good exercise, it's enjoyable and it will increase his chances of survival in an accident in the water. Note the following:

- Avoid public swimming pools until your baby is six months old.

- Children's swimming classes are a good idea if you do not feel confident teaching your child yourself. Baby classes are usually held in special pools where the water is warmer and where additional hygiene precautions are taken. Contact your local pool or the Amateur Swimming Association for details.

- Keep your baby moving all the time in the water so that he stays warm.

- Special nappies are available for use in the water – ordinary ones become waterlogged and uncomfortable.

- Always use inflatable armbands or floats specially designed for babies, even if you are with them in the pool.

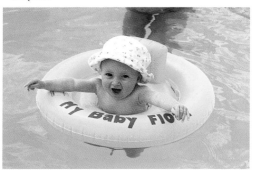

Teething and caring for teeth

At around six months old your baby will get the first of twenty milk teeth. This can cause soreness in the gums, and general grumpiness and fractiousness, dribbling, a slightly raised temperature, and looser bowels. Massaging his gums with a cooled finger, and giving him something to gnaw on will help. Teething is one of the greatest causes of sleepless nights for babies and parents. If there is much discomfort, calendula granules or a teething preparation can be applied to the gums or Calpol (baby paracetamol) can be used as directed on the label.

Clean your baby's gums and the early teeth as soon as they start to appear, using a soft toothbrush and a tiny amount of toothpaste – no larger than half a pea. Let him do it himself from around 18 months. Avoid sugar in food if he is eating solids, and do not dip a dummy into sugar water or honey, or give sugar-rich drinks in the bottle. Never let your baby go to sleep with a bottle, because this will encourage bacteria to grow in the mouth overnight.

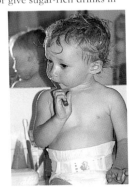

Make caring for teeth a fun part of your child's healthcare routine as he grows up. Change his toothbrush every few months or more often if there is a cold or other infection. Regular brushing along with a sensible diet should keep tooth decay and plaque at bay. Disclosing agents will show any plaque left behind. Some dentists may also recommend that a fluoride supplement in the form of drops or tablets is used in areas where there is inadequate fluoride in the water supply.

Keep sugar as an occasional treat in your older child's diet, and make sure he has plenty of Vitamin D and calcium-rich foods to strengthen growing teeth (and bones). Encourage regular six-monthly visits to the dentist once teeth have started to come through, so that your child does not develop a fear of this as he grows older. You can register him with a dentist under the NHS as soon as he is born; NHS dental treatment for children is free.

If your child falls and hits his teeth, take him to a dentist. Sometimes the teeth will darken or fall out but this should not affect the growth of second teeth later.

Temper tantrums

Although all children are capable of tantrums, these seem to peak around the age of two. They can involve shouting, crying, stamping feet, screaming, kicking, rolling on the ground, holding the breath and throwing things. These outbursts can be frightening for parents and children alike. Often they are over in a few minutes, but they can sometimes last for up to an hour at a time, and some children have them daily. Mostly, however, they flare up only occasionally, and usually at home with parents or a main carer.

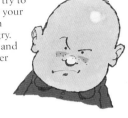

Prevention is always best: try to ensure a regular routine for your child which keeps him from becoming too tired or hungry. Learn to recognize triggers and stressful situations and either avoid them or prepare for them as well as possible. Often distraction will be enough to head off a tantrum.

Try to remain calm and be as reassuring as possible and, most of all, don't lose your temper. If it is too trying, you should leave the room – first making sure that your child is in no physical danger. With younger children, a loud noise or an unusual activity (such as you beginning to dance) will shock them out of their behaviour, and allow you to comfort them and return to everyday activities.

Don't be tempted to bribe your child out of a tantrum, or to give in to one, as this will only set a negative precedent for you both.

If tantrums occur outside the home, such as in a supermarket or when visiting, leave straight away, or take yourselves to a quiet corner where your child has to focus on you and you on him. Use plenty of eye-contact, and be prepared to take some time to settle before continuing with whatever it was you were doing. Try to talk to your child about his tantrums when you are both calm.

Temperature

Taking your child's temperature is easiest if you place a thermometer under his armpit, or use a forehead strip that will give a visual readout. A young child will tend to resist you placing the thermometer in his mouth, and find it hard to leave it there for any length of time. There is also the possibility that he will bite down on it.

Feel your child's forehead and if it is warm to the touch, and he shows signs of feverishness, then check his temperature. If he is old enough to have the thermometer placed in his mouth, the normal reading will be 37° C (98.6° F). If you are using the axillary temperature (under the armpit), keep the thermometer in place for about three minutes, and do something to distract your child's attention so that you can keep him still for that long. Wipe the armpit dry before placing the thermometer there, and hold it in place by keeping that arm flat against your child's side. Normal readings for underarm temperatures are 36.4° C (97.6° F). You can also take a rectal temperature, but this is not always recommended, and if your child is too sick and restless to allow you to take a forehead, mouth or underarm temperature, then you need to contact your doctor.

Your child will display a range of temperature changes as he grows up. Things like high activity levels, excitement and allergies will all cause immediate and short-lived rises in temperature. If your child is generally excitable, introduce 'quiet times' to soothe him.

If your child becomes flushed and develops a raised temperature after eating or drinking, it may be that he has an allergy to a particular foodstuff or additive. The most common sensitivities are to chemical preservatives and flavourings and to orange food dyes. Eliminating these from the diet should be sufficient to restore calm to the system, but if you suspect an allergy to a food or food group, such as dairy products or wheat, then work with a professional to remove them, and balance the diet effectively.

> **Caution:** A raised temperature combined with other symptoms means your child is in need of care. Consult your doctor or the hospital if your child has a temperature above 38° C (100.4° F) and is unusually drowsy or lethargic, is not feeding, is fractious and crying, or has vomiting or diarrhoea. If your baby is less than three months old, contact your doctor straight away in all cases of fever.

See also **Fever**

Thumb-sucking

Thumb- or finger-sucking can be very comforting to a young child. Parents often worry that the habit will stick, or that it will cause damage to the emerging

teeth, but it does not affect a child's first teeth.
Children often put things into their mouth for
comfort, and to quiet the sucking reflex. Most children
will grow out of thumb-sucking quite naturally, and
well before it is likely to cause any harm to second
teeth, which generally begin to emerge around the age
of six. If you are concerned or this habit seems to be
going on for too long, some simple strategies can be
most effective; rather than making an issue of thumb-
sucking, try to divert your child's attention from it:

- give him something else to do with his hands;
- hold his hand, or engage him in some dextrous
  activity;
- introduce older children to manicuring skills and
  hand care;
- introduce a system (a star chart for example) where-
  by your child is rewarded for not sucking his thumb
  for extended periods.

See also **Comfort behaviours, Dummies**

Toys

Toys are invaluable educational aids, and will provide
stimulus and relaxation to your child, as well as
developing his ability to function separately from you.

It is never too early to make a strong link between
enjoyment and learning. Your baby's first toys are likely

to be tactile, like teddies or rag dolls, and a mobile of some sort that will encourage his focusing skills and attention. Make sure first toys are not big or loud enough to be scary. Soon, anything that squeaks or buzzes, flashes lights or moves will engage your child's natural inquisitiveness and his delight in new things.

It is important for children to be introduced to a range of toys and activities:

- Make sure that the toys you choose for your child are safe and appropriate for his age. Never let your baby or young child play with anything that could be pushed into a nose or ear, or swallowed.

- Avoid toys with small parts for children under three, and look for a guarantee on all toys indicating that they meet British or other relevant safety standards.

- From around four months your child will find rattles and similar toys entertaining.

- Balls and ball games improve mobility and hand–eye co-ordination, as well as encouraging activity.

- Board games enhance vocabulary and conversational skills as well as teaching about team-work and competition.

- Dolls and teddies encourage children to articulate emotion and develop their caring side.

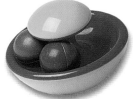

- Older children will enjoy games that can be played on their own and with others, and that have rules that will help them learn about structure and discipline, as well as about relationships with others.

Sharing toys is a wonderful opportunity to enhance social skills. Always monitor your child's toys, including those they receive as gifts – you may prefer, for example that they don't play with toy guns or weapons.

Your child may develop a special or favourite toy, teddy, book or game. This is fine, and you can encourage his interest by making sure you include his special toy for as long as this attraction lasts. Be sensitive to any such attachment and do not try to get your child to share, leave, or give away a 'special' toy before he is ready to do so.

Once a week, wrap small enough soft toys in a plastic bag and place in the freezer overnight to kill off house dust mites, and wash soft toys and balls.

See also **Hand–eye co-ordination, Manual skills**

Travel sickness

Travel sickness is thought to result from an upset in the delicate balance mechanism in the inner ear, caused by motion. Simple measures will often help.

Travelling by car:

- Make sure there is enough air in the car by opening one of the front windows.

- Regulate the temperature, ensuring it is not too hot or stifling.

- Keep the atmosphere calm by encouraging quiet activities or rest while travelling.

- Try not to let your child become too excited before the journey.

- Wearing a Travel Band may help older children. This is a simple band, available from chemists, that is worn around the wrist and has a plastic or metal stud sewn into it. When worn correctly, this applies gentle pressure on an acupressure point in the wrist and will soothe any nausea.

Travelling by air:

- Tell the cabin crew that your child suffers from travel sickness as they are usually experienced in diversionary tactics.

- Babies will be comforted, especially through take-off and landing, if you can feed them.

- Older children will often be diverted by interesting activities within the cabin, or if they can help spot other planes on the runway or clouds nearby.

- 'Popping' or painful ears – particularly during take-off and landing – may be helped by sucking or chewing.

Travelling by sea:

- Sit on deck (weather permitting) with plenty of access to fresh air.
- Encourage a little walk every half hour or so.
- Discourage young children from running around and becoming too excited.

If your child is physically sick, give him a sweet-tasting drink to wash his mouth with if he cannot brush his teeth. Sit quietly with him and rest. Often vomiting will mark an end to the feelings of nausea. Give your child plenty to drink, and only light foods or fruit until he feels more settled. Avoid making more of an isolated incident than is necessary, so that your child will not automatically associate future travel with sickness.

See also **Car journeys**

Twins

One in 80 pregnancies is a multiple pregnancy. In 1996, nearly 10,000 sets of twins were born in the UK, 300 sets of triplets, and 9 sets of quadruplets or more. The likelihood of a woman having twins increases as she grows older. There is also a strong genetic link, so if twins run in your family, your chances of having them are higher.

Twins (or more) do require a little more planning and preparation than a single birth in practical terms, and buying two of everything from cots and highchairs to car seats can make for considerable extra expense.

Identical twins will have a very strong connection to one another. Very early in life this can mean that they both want to feed at the same time, and both cry at the same time, and so on. However, it is possible to feed both at the same time, and if you are bottle-feeding you can share feeding with a partner or helper.

Keeping to a routine will help to provide some structure when coping with twins, and it is very important to establish a good support network early on. **Post-natal depression** (*see* page 139) is more likely with multiple births, but this can often be because of the additional workload, stress, and lack of support. As parents of twins you may be able to get a home help from your local council, depending on their policy. If not, ask your health visitor for suggestions.

Even identical twins will have some differentiating physical features or ways of doing things, and it is important to each child's development that you address them separately, and value their individuality and uniqueness.

Twins' development rates are often different from that of single children, and it is quite normal for them to develop at different rates from one another too, and for their speech to develop rather later than in other children. This is because they often have their own private methods of communicating with each other.

See also **Breast-feeding**

Urinary tract infections

Cystitis is an infection of the bladder. It can occur at any age, and is much more common in girls than in boys because their urine outlet tube is shorter, making it easier for infections to travel up to the bladder. Any part of the urinary system may become affected, including the kidneys, so it is important to have it treated as early as possible.

Symptoms usually include soreness on passing urine, a frequent desire to go to the toilet and a slight fever. There may also be discomfort in the lower abdomen.

Treat by giving plenty of water and lemon barley water to drink. Sit the child in a bath of warm water to which a teaspoon of salt has been added to relieve pain on urination. When dry, place a warm hot water bottle on the lower back, and encourage plenty of rest. Cranberry juice can be a useful remedy but may be difficult to take without added sugar so it is not recommended for babies or very young children.

Toilet hygiene is very important. Teach your children to wipe from front to back to avoid any contamination by faecal germs (this also applies to cleaning a child in nappies), and always to wash their hands after using the toilet. Regular bathing will help.

If symptoms persist for more than a few hours, or worsen, and include low back pain, contact your doctor straight away. A urine sample will usually be taken, and a course of antibiotics may well be prescribed.

Vaccinations

One of the first major decisions you will need to take about your child's health may be whether or not to have him vaccinated. Medical evidence is clear that before routine vaccination and our current levels of hygiene, childhood diseases killed and maimed alarmingly high numbers of children. Also, the risks associated with vaccinations are negligible in relation to possible death or disability from the disease, and to the possible benefits to society of eradicating or greatly limiting these diseases.

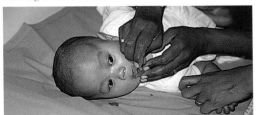

Consult with your GP before making your final decision, and consider the following:

- the state of your own and your partner's immunity to infection – this will have a profound impact on your child's;
- whether you breast-feed – this will transfer your immunity to your baby;

DISEASE	TIME
Diphtheria, tetanus, and whooping cough (pertussis). DTP or triple vaccine	Injections at 2, 3, and 4 months. Diphtheria and tetanus are repeated at 4–5 years old.
Polio	Oral vaccine at 2, 3 and 4 months, repeated at 4–5 years old.
Measles, mumps and rubella (German measles). MMR	Injection at 12–18 months.
Haemophilus influenza type b HiB, HiB meningitis, epiglottis, septicaemia, septic arthritis, osteomyelitis, pneumonia	Injection at 2, 3 and 4 months, or just one injection for child over 1 year old

- whether there is any history of malreaction in either of your families.

Your baby is likely to be offered a series of vaccinations against polio, diphtheria, tetanus and whooping cough, measles, mumps and rubella and haemophilus infections, including a form of meningitis (HiB vaccine) given at various stages and intervals.

REACTION	PROTECTION OFFERED
Child may become feverish and the site of the injection may be sore	Tetanus must be repeated every 10 years for continued protection
Reactions are not recorded	Has to be repeated every 10 years for continued protection
Child may become feverish and have a slight rash	Not known how long protection lasts
Site of injection may become red and swollen	After 4 years old the child should have developed a natural resistance and does not need to be vaccinated again.

These are usually injected into the arm or thigh, and your baby will need more than one injection, or a booster. Polio is given as drops. In some parts of the UK, vaccinations for meningococcal meningitis are now routinely available for babies and teenagers. Ask your GP for advice.

See also **Fever, Measles, Meningitis, Mumps, Rubella, Whooping cough**

Vomiting

Vomiting is the quickest way for your child's system to eject something it doesn't like. Triggers may be:

- unwanted or unhealthy food or drink, which is expelled quickly and often suddenly, and then the episode will be over;

- movement and overheating;

- travel or motion sickness;

- children becoming over-excited;

- migraines, or more serious concerns such as appendicitis or meningitis.

Babies will often 'posset' or regurgitate a little after a feed, but this is usually clear or milky, and causes no discomfort. It is a result of taking in air with their feed, and usually stops when they are about six months old and are spending more time upright.

If your child has an episode of vomiting, put him to bed with a clean container nearby for him to use if he feels he is going to be sick again. Give him frequent small sips of water, diluted fruit juice, or water to which has been added a pinch of salt and a teaspoon of sugar. Take your time over reintroducing solid foods, and keep an eye on his temperature. Usually your child will show you he is feeling better by his desire to be up and active again.

Consult your doctor if vomiting continues for more than a few hours, or in the case of a baby if there are repeated episodes. Your doctor must also be called in cases of projectile vomiting (when milk or food is violently vomited up straight after a feed).

Caution: Consult your doctor straight away if vomiting is accompanied by any or all of the following: earache, high fever, sharp abdominal pain, a rash, rigidity or aversion to light. These are all indications of more serious concerns.

See also **Travel sickness**

Walking

Babies may start to walk at any stage from ten months on. Some children walk earlier than others, and some will be content to shuffle around on their bottoms for many months yet. Early attempts can be encouraged.

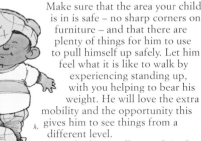

Make sure that the area your child is in is safe – no sharp corners on furniture – and that there are plenty of things for him to use to pull himself up safely. Let him feel what it is like to walk by experiencing standing up, with you helping to bear his weight. He will love the extra mobility and the opportunity this gives him to see things from a different level.

Push-along trolleys and similar toys are useful for a baby who's learning to walk. Stairs will take a little longer to master and will probably be taken slowly with both feet on each step (not alternating) until he is older.

See also **Crawling, Shoes**

Weaning

Some babies are extremely hungry and will need to start 'solids' sooner rather than later. Four months is the earliest, but many babies do not start before six months. Breast- or bottle-feeding can continue alongside solid food, and if both you and your baby enjoy it there is no reason to stop. It also ensures a reliable source of nutrients while your child is experimenting with new and different foods. When you are ready to start weaning your baby, try teaching him to use a lidded feeding cup for milk or cooled, boiled water. (You can start this from around four months.) Always give solids first, then offer a cup of milk or water. You can offer the breast or bottle as well, but gradually cut down, or if it works better you can cut out the breast or bottle altogether at one feed a day, offering the cup instead.

As weaning progresses, supplement your baby's fluid intake (but not with sweetened drinks). Eventually the breast/bottle will be used for comforting rather than nutritional purposes so you must ensure his diet is balanced.

With gradual weaning your breasts should return more or less to their pre-pregnancy size and shape, with minimal discomfort. Consult your GP if you experience any breast pain for longer than a week.

See also **Breast-feeding, First foods**

Whooping cough

This usually begins with flu-like symptoms – sneezing, mild coughing, runny nose, fever and aching limbs. The 'whoop' is a distinctive sound made as your child gulps in air after each coughing fit. These can be severe, and may lead to vomiting. Symptoms, especially the cough, are usually worst at night. Whooping cough can be very serious in babies under one year old. It is easily spread through airborne droplets. Incubation can be between one and three weeks, and the ailment itself can last for as long as three months. It is usual nowadays to vaccinate against it.

Home treatment involves keeping your child warm and well rested, with lots to drink. If he vomits, give him a small snack after each expulsion, because he will be most likely to keep the food down then. Keep a bowl to hand for him to spit into, and this will help keep his lungs as clear as possible. Keep the child out of contact with others as much as possible, and always let other parents and carers know if there is whooping cough in the house.

> **Caution:** Newborn babies and premature babies are particularly at risk from whooping cough. Always consult your GP if whooping cough is suspected, and complications such as pneumonia and dehydration can be monitored.

See also **Vaccinations**

Worms

The most common intestinal worm infestation is the threadworm. The eggs of these can be picked up on unwashed fruit and vegetables that have been contaminated, and will hatch and grow within a month. The symptoms are itching around the anus, and the thread-like worms can sometimes be seen in the stools or around the anus. With heat, lots of sugar in the diet, or a large infestation, the irritation can be enormous, and scratching can lead to areas of broken skin all around the bottom. If the bottom is scratched, and then hands are placed in or near the mouth, the whole cycle will be repeated.

Toxocara worm can be picked up from contaminated dog or cat faeces, and this is particularly dangerous for pregnant women and infants. This worm works its way into the bloodstream and the symptoms include loss of appetite, abdominal pain and fever.

Children must be taught to wash their hands before and after eating, going to the bathroom, touching soil, etc., and care must be taken to stop younger infants rolling in areas where animals have fouled. Make sure any food you give them has been washed.

Worm medication can be obtained over the counter from your pharmacist, but check that the preparation is specifically designed for children. Also make sure that the whole family is treated. Threadworm eggs can live in bedding for up to three weeks, so a thorough spring clean is advisable.

Useful addresses

Association of Breast-feeding Mothers
PO Box 441, St Albans
Herts AL4 0AS
Tel: 020-8778 4769

Association for Post-Natal Illness
25 Jerdan Place
London SW6 1BE
Tel: 020-7386 0868

Foundation for the Study of Infant Deaths
14 Halkin Street
London SW1X 7DP
Tel: 020-7235 0965

Hyperactive Children's Support Group
71 Whyke Lane
Chichester, PO19 2LD
Tel: 01903-725182

The Informed Parent
19 Woodlands Road
Harrow HA1 2RT
Tel: 020-8861 1022

Institute of Complementary Medicine
PO Box 194
London SE16 1QZ
Tel: 020-7237 5165

Osteopathic Centre for Children (OCC)
19a Cavendish Square
Harcourt House
London W1M 9AD
Tel: 020-7495 1231

Parents at Work
45 Beech Street
London EC2Y 8AD
Tel: 020-7628 3565

TAMBA (Twins and Multiple Births Association)
Harnott House
309 Chester Road
Little Sutton
South Wirral L66 1QQ
Tel: 0870-121 4000

COLLINS GEM
BABIES'
names

COLLINS GEM
BEER

COLLINS GEM
BIRDS

COLLINS GEM
CALORIE
Counter

COLLINS GEM
FACT FILE

COLLINS GEM
FENG SHUI

COLLINS GEM
FLAGS

COLLINS GEM
Healthy
EATING

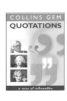
COLLINS GEM
QUOTATIONS

COLLINS GEM
SAS
Self-Defence

COLLINS GEM
SAS
Survival Guide

COLLINS GEM
SEASHORE

COLLINS GEM
TREES

COLLINS GEM
Understanding
DREAMS

COLLINS GEM
WILD
flowers

COLLINS GEM
WINE
Dictionary